Racing Among the Ages

A Crowdsourcing Approach to Age-Grading the 5K

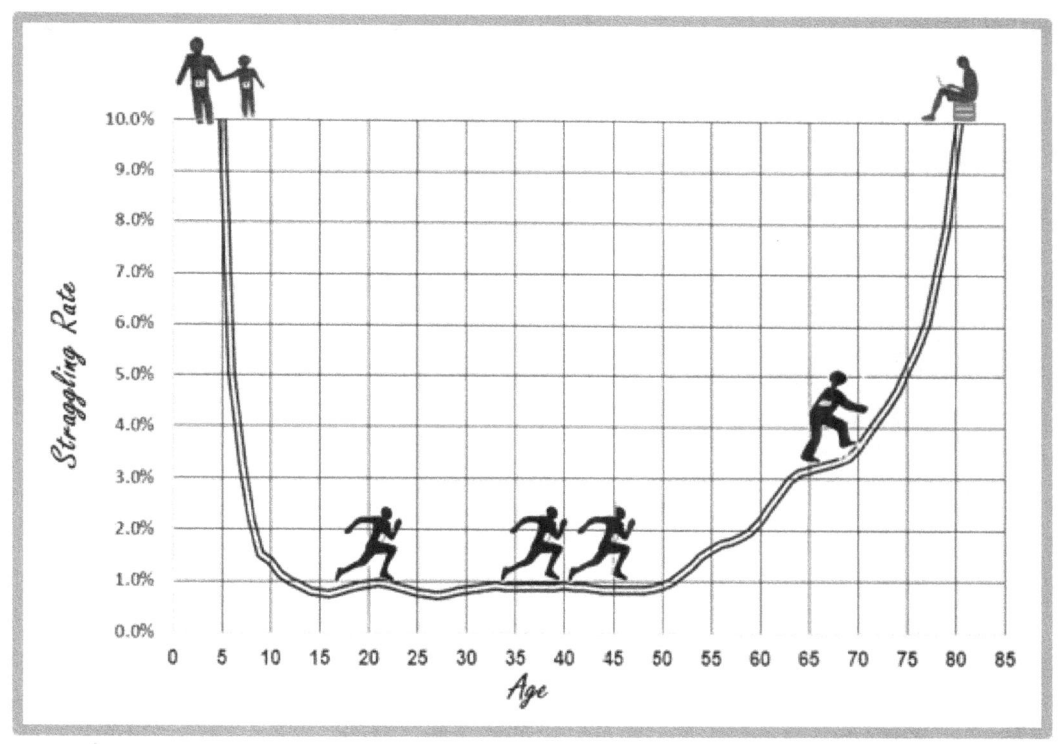

Includes Detailed Centile Tables

David P. Dyer, Ph.D.

Racing among the Ages
A Crowdsourcing Approach to Age-Grading the 5K

David P. Dyer

ISBN-13: 978-1519350428

ISBN-10: 1519350422

> The race is not to the swift, nor the battle to the strong . . . but time and chance happen to them all.
>
> Ecclesiastes 9:11

CONTENTS

Abstract

Age-grading metrics are used to compare the performances of athletes of different ages. They are also used to compare athletes of differing gender. However, data collected from almost thirteen hundred 5K races and over one million individual race records demonstrate that current age-grading methodology – derived from world records – does not apply to the overwhelming majority of running athletes.

In this text, I propose and then develop in detail an improved methodology for age grading that is based on Participation Corrected Centiles (PCC). An analysis of the extreme variations seen in age specific participation rates leads to the resolution of technical issues which have heretofore limited the use of percentiles for age-grading endurance races. In comparison to current age-grading methodologies, the approach described here is both more accurate and more credible.

Extensive tables are included which allow athletes to determine their age specific percentiles and to compare their performances with all other 5K participants.

1. Introduction

Age is a powerful determinant of athletic performance. Young athletes expect their running speed to improve with each passing year. In spite of their best efforts, aging athletes will eventually slow down; and as time and chance take their toll, some aging athletes will put away their racing shoes for the last time and only watch from the sidelines.

But the desire to compete remains strong and endures even as other abilities decline. This point was brought home several years ago as I was visiting a relative in a nursing home. Around the perimeter of large room, two very elderly gentlemen using walkers were locked in a deadly serious slow motion duel. The leader smiled with the confidence of a winner as he looked around the room to see who was watching this contest. The other gentleman was totally focused as he matched the leader step for step, his intensity would have done credit to any Olympic runner determined not to settle for silver.

In recognition of the effect of age and of the desire to compete against our peers, many 5K (and other endurance) races divide participants into 5 year (or 10 year) age groups so that each participant competes directly with only individuals of approximately the same age. A very young and a very old runner can place well within their respective age groups, even if it is unlikely that they will be among overall leaders.

However, smaller races will have very few or even a single participant in some age groups; how can the performance of these individuals be evaluated? A 60 year old woman is running slower than she did at 30, but for her age is she now doing better or worse? A father (age 36) and his son (age 14) both run a 5K race in 25 minutes; for their age, who performed the best?

To answer questions such as these, various methodologies collectively known as "age grading" have been developed. A number of websites offer age grading calculators; for example:

http://www.howardgrubb.co.uk/athletics/wmalookup15.html

http://www.mastersathletics.net/index.php?id=2595

http://www.heartbreakhill.org/age_graded.htm

For endurance races, all of these calculators are built in reference to the World Masters Athletics (WMA, formerly WAVA) age standards, but differ slightly depending on whether they use the standards set in 2015, 2006/10, or 1994. All are based on using world records to estimate the current upper limit (age standard) for human performance at each age. New world records are one of the primary reasons the age standards are periodically updated. More information on the methodology used to develop these types of age standards can be found in Fair (2007, 1994), Jones (2015), Sterken (2003), Grubb (1998), and Reece and Finnessy (2014). I will use the 2015 factors when I refer to the WMA age standards.

With these calculators, an individual can compare his or her performance to the age standard. For example, using the first calculator listed above (WMA Age-grading calculator 2015, 5kmRoad), the age standard for a 43 year old man in a 5K race is 14 minutes. If he runs a 5K in 20 minutes, he is (14/20) = 70% as fast as the age standard. Two individuals of differing ages can compare their age performance percentages to see who had the best age graded performance.

In spite of the ready availability of age standards and age grading methodology, it has had limited application in actual races and is poorly understood (if known at all) by many race participants. Since many or even most races employ computer technology, computational issues should not be a deterrent. Among race directors there may be some hesitation to adopt "new" procedures since the status quo seems to be working just fine. However, among the reasons that current approaches to age grading have not (and should not) gain more widespread application is that they simply do not work very well for any but the most elite athletes.

There are two issues with current approaches. The first issue is that standards developed from world records are not generally applicable to the great majority of running (and walking) athletes. Modeling world records and the upper limits of human performance is an interesting exercise in itself. And it is certainly deserving of the great effort and sophisticated statistical modeling it currently enjoys. However, for those who wish to index the performance of all athletes using models developed for world class athletes, the elephant in the room is the assumption that average athletes and the super elite change at the same rate with age. R. C. Fair (2007) has pointed out that this is a key limitation of any age grading approach that is based solely on best performance records.

Certainly, even if a perfect standard based on world class performances did exist, there is no reason to expect it to be useful in the "real world" of everyday 5K races. And in spite of the understandable human desire for reification, the data presented here show that applying any single standard across a wide range of abilities can do more harm than good.

A second issue with using current age standards is confusion between the meaning of "percent of an age standard" and "performance percentile". Standardized academic tests are often evaluated on a percentile basis. For example, someone in the 90th percentile scored better than 90% of his or her peers. So it is natural to incorrectly assume that WMA age graded percents can be interpreted as percentiles. The third age grading calculator above (Heartbreak Hill: Boston Striders) possibly adds to this confusion by mistakenly using the term "percentile" in reference to age grading using a percent of a standard. With this calculator, a 38 year old female running a 5K in 20 minutes is given an "achievement percentile" of 74% even though the data presented here shows her performance would place her ahead of more than 99% of other same age female participants! In a recent article on how to use age graders, John Davis (2015) points out that the output of current age grading calculators are frequently confused with percentiles and even suggests that percentiles might be more meaningful. He also lists other problems with the approach used by current age grading calculators.

A possible resolution for all of these issues may be to simply age grade race performance using <u>actual</u> percentiles. As we shall see, this approach works quite well, <u>provided</u> we take into account the participation censoring that occurs for the very youngest and very oldest individuals and also the variation in the single year population sizes among the different ages.

2. The Data

The data consists of 1,042,126 U.S. 5K road race records from the years 2008 through 2014. Forty-eight states and D.C are represented. California, Massachusetts, New York, and Illinois had the most participants in this data set and Idaho and Wyoming had none. The data collection process consisted of searching for 5K races and "trots" using various search engines such as Google or Yahoo, as well as more specialized sites such as "Running in the USA" (www.runningintheusa.com/), "RunWashington" (www.runwashington.com/), and "Fleet Feet Sports" (e.g. www.fleetfeetstlouis.com). Once a 5K race was found, the results were downloaded -- provided the formatting used by the web site allowed a relatively easy conversion to my standard format. No races with less than 100 total participants were included and races with less than 400 participants were included with lower probability because the download effort required per participant was relatively high for these small races and because small races were more likely to have a non-standard data format. If both chip and gun times were available, the chip time was used.

Only races open to both males and females and all ages 5 and over were included. Within this group of races, the highest time recorded was 1 hour 59 minutes and 18 seconds. The lowest time recorded was 13 minutes and 26 seconds. By way of comparison, as of June 2015, ARRS recorded the world record for road 5K's at 12 minutes and 59.5 seconds (http://www.arrs.net/SA_R5K.htm).

The majority of races allowed at least one hour for participants to complete the course. More than 75% of participants were in races where the slowest time recorded was over one hour. Similarly 91% of participants were in races with a slowest time of over 55 minutes and 97% were in races with a slowest time of more than 50 minutes. Recognizing that the time of the slowest recorded participant is necessarily less than the race cut off time suggests that over 75% to 97% of participants had at least one hour, if they needed it.

With a net total of 1283 races, the average race size was 812 participants. Because of the intentional exclusion of the smallest races, the average race size here is somewhat larger than the overall average of all U.S. races during the years in question. Nevertheless, the gross race statistics here are reasonably comparable to those reported by Running USA for 2011 (the middle year of this study). I found 45% males and 55% females, Running USA found 43% and 57% respectively. The median time for males was 28:03, Running USA found 28:05. The median time for females was 33:27, Running USA found 34:09. See www.runningusa.org/State-of-Sport-Road-Race-Trends.

Prior to use, the data were subjected to several audits. Seven races were excluded because of discrepancies in reporting chip versus gun times.

Within each of the remaining 1283 races, the five year age/gender group winners were identified and then subjected to a review by name if their speed exceeded the mean of the corresponding age group by more than three standard deviations. Similarly, any individual with a speed more than a set number of standard deviations above his or her single year age/gender group mean was also reviewed by name. (The set number of standard deviations varied between 1.6 and 3.9, depending on the total number of individuals of that age and gender). Somewhat surprisingly, most individuals identified as having an extremely high speed were confirmed as legitimate by results from other races or by press releases identifying them as a former Olympian, a former state cross country champion, a US age group record holder for another distance, etc. A total of 88 individual extreme race records were excluded for such things as a wrong age, a lack of any other record of significant running accomplishment, or the timing service obviously got information in the wrong columns.

3. Methods and Terminology

3.1 Methods: Centiles

Unlike standards developed from best performance records, this study looks at the entire distribution of race performances from slowest to fastest. Consequently centiles (i.e. percentiles) are used as the measure of performance: an individual's performance can be expressed as a centile of his or her single year age and gender group.

For any single year age and gender group, the performances were ranked and the rank, R, corresponding to the Pth centile was calculated as R = 0.5+P*N, where N is the number of individuals in the group. If R was an integer, then the speed of the individual with this rank is the speed corresponding to the Pth centile; otherwise the Pth centile speed is interpolated between the speeds of the two closest ranked individuals (Schoonjans et. al., 2011). For example, if there were 10,000 participants in an age/gender group, then the 90th centile is the midpoint between the speeds of the $9,000^{th}$ and $9,001^{th}$ individuals.

3.2 Methods: Smoothing

A nine point, cubic Savitzky-Golay filter (Schafer, 2011; Savitzky and Golay, 1964) was applied twice in succession when data smoothing would add clarity. This filter uses a local least squares polynomial approximation to estimate the speed at each age.

Since a nine-point cubic polynomial cannot be centered on the four oldest (or four youngest) ages in a series, these endpoints were smoothed using a seven point quadratic polynomial ending on the oldest (or starting on the youngest) age in the series.

3.3 Methods: Participation Rates

To standardize participation rates, I used U.S. census information for Annual Estimates of the Resident Population by Single Year of Age and Sex for the United States: July 1, 2011 (https://www.census.gov/popest/). For 5K race data collected in years other than 2011, the relevant population was estimated using the appropriate age offset. (e.g., 30 year old participants in 2013 races were pared against the population of 28 year olds in 2011). Since participation rates at each age are based on the living population size, the effect of mortality is factored out.

The estimate by Running USA (http://www.runningusa.org) of the annual total number (8,300,000) of 5K race finishers was used to calculate the age related standardized participation rates. For example, in the data collected here, 1.35% of the participants were 40 year old females. During the time period covered by this study, the weighted average resident population of 40 year old females was 2,068,266. Consequently, the standardized race participation rate was 0.0135*8,300,000/2,068,266 = 0.0542 or 54.2 per 1000 population. (Note: since the estimated annual total number of participants is only used as a common scaling factor, primarily for display purposes, the accuracy of the calculated centiles and participation rate adjustments are independent of the 8,300,000 estimate of annual finishers).

3.4 Methods: Life Stages

For present purposes four life stages are defined as follows:

> Child: 5-11 years
> Adolescent: 12-24 years
> Adult: 25-39 years
> Masters: 40 years & over

Several organizations understand the terminology "Adolescent" as used here to encompass both adolescents and young adults. For example, the CDC and NIHCM (National Institute for Health Care Management) identify young adults as 19-24 year olds and the US Dept. of health and Human Services lists young adults as 20-24 year olds. The Masters Age range is consistent with the USA Track and Field Long Distance Running category (www.usatf.org/groups/Masters/). The variables measured here (speed, participation rates, and straggling rates) show distinct patterns in each of these life stages.

4. Results

4.1 Results: Participation Rates

Within current popular culture and for a wide variety of athletic events, there is a vigorous and ongoing debate about awarding trophies and recognition to either those who excelled in an event or, alternatively, to all participants. An inherent purpose of age grading is to identify the best and the winners across all ages, so the whole mechanism associated with age grading comes down squarely on the side of recognizing excellence and winners. However, at the extremes of age, completing a 5K race in approximately an hour becomes so difficult and so rare, that the terms "participant" and "winner" appear to gradually merge into a single concept.

Age related changes in participation rates are dramatic. For example, in the Masters stage, between ages 40 and 89, the male participation rate declined by a factor of 52 and the female participation rate declined by a massive factor of 468. By contrast, during this period, the uncorrected (raw) median speed of both male and female participants declined by less than a factor of two. Since the participation rates are calculated on the basis of the living population at each age, the changes in participation rates are <u>not</u> a reflection of age related mortality.

Figure 1 shows the very large range in participation rates. Both males and females show similar patterns. The participation rate curves show three major features: (1) a rapid increase during Childhood, (2) a dip and then rebound during Adolescence, (3) a leveling off (Males) or slow decline (Females) during the Adult stage, and finally (4), in the Masters stage, a relentless and exponential decline. [Note: for the Masters stage, a plot of the log of the participation rates vs. age confirm the rate of decline is actually somewhat faster than exponential!]

Specific turning points are identified in Figures 2A and 2B which show the 2nd derivative of the previously described Savitzky-Golay smoothing filter. The extrema of the 2nd derivative identify the ages when the gradient of the participation curve achieves a local extreme amount of change.

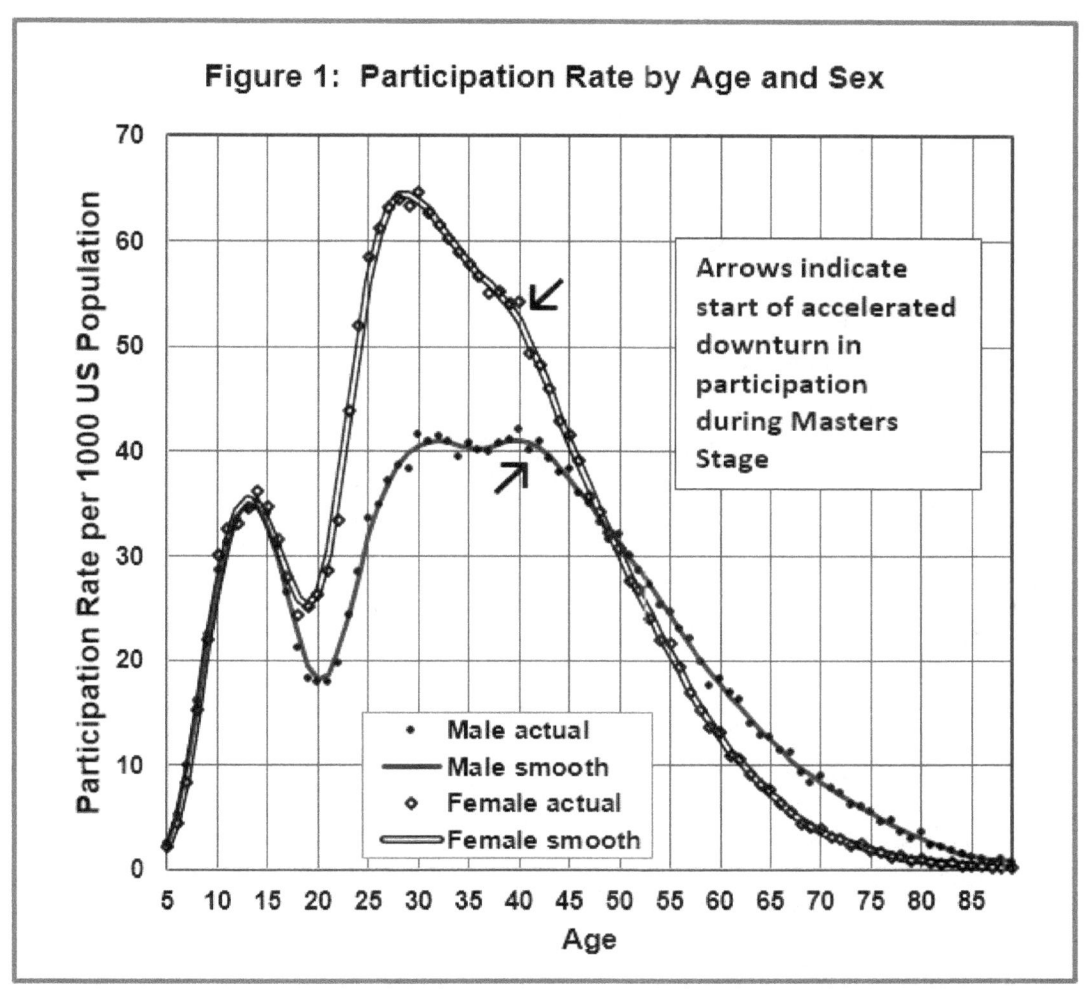

For example, for females, the decline in participation rates accelerates markedly at age 40. For males this acceleration occurs at age 42.

Age related changes in participation rates depend on three trends: (1) the number of new active participants just starting out or returning to racing, (2) the number becoming inactive and dropping out, and (3) how frequently active runners (joggers/walkers) are able to participate. How we interpret the speed centiles in light of large differences in age related participation rates depends directly on the causes of the changes in participation rates.

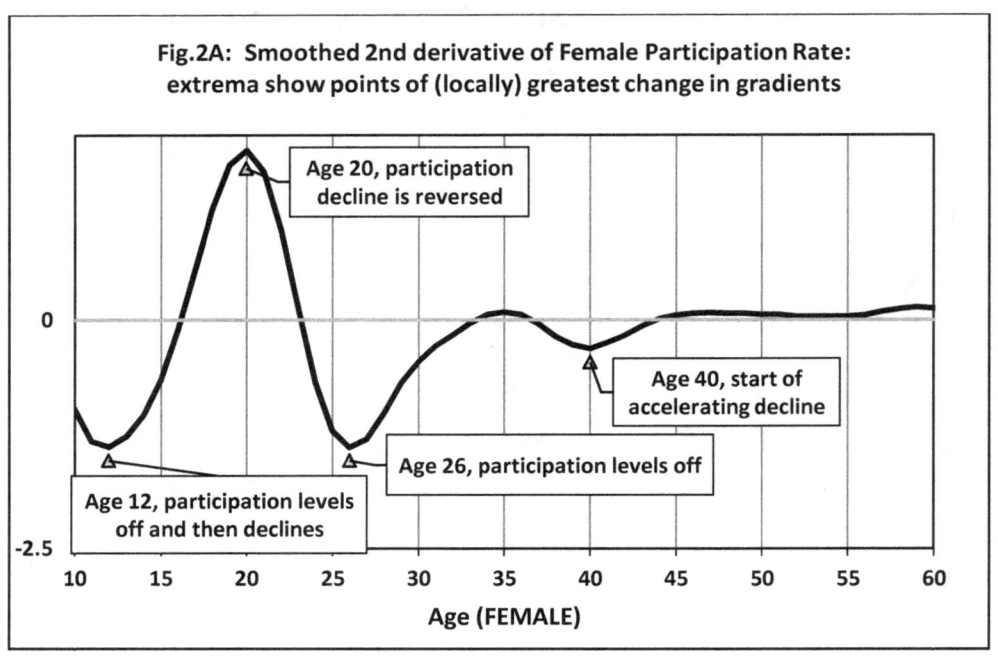

Fig.2A: Smoothed 2nd derivative of Female Participation Rate: extrema show points of (locally) greatest change in gradients

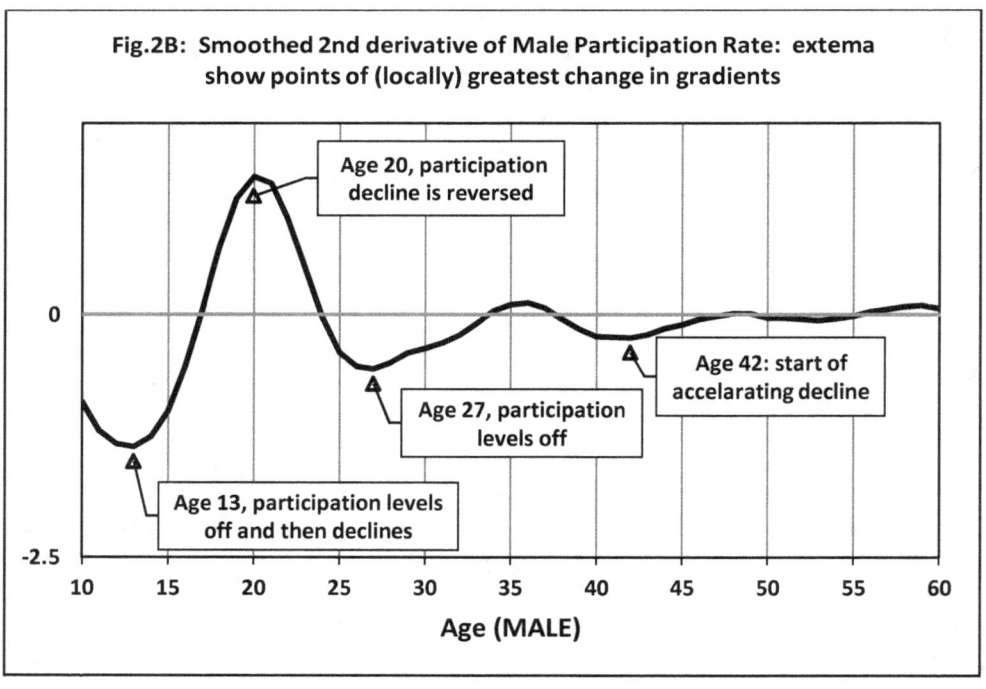

Fig.2B: Smoothed 2nd derivative of Male Participation Rate: extema show points of (locally) greatest change in gradients

If changes in participation rates are uncorrelated with performance, then no adjustment in the speed centiles is needed. For example, suppose between an earlier age and a later age, a number of individuals stop participating but that these drop outs proportionately represent all ability levels. In this case, a runner in the earlier age would perform at the same centile among both all participants and also among the participants who would not later drop out.

On the other hand, if changes in participation rates are closely correlated with performance ability, then adjustments in the calculated centiles may be necessary to insure an apples to apples comparison. For example, suppose only the slowest half of the participants drop out between a younger age and an older age. In this case, a runner who was faster than 75% of all participants in the earlier age would only be faster than 50% of those who would not later drop out.

The dip and then recovery in participation rates during the adolescent/young adult life stage occurs simultaneously with a number of major life events: teen social development, high school graduation, college, a first full time job, getting married, moving to a new location, etc. We might suppose that both faster and slower individuals are similarly at risk to be pulled away from racing by these unrelated competing life events. During the Adult stage, the number of dependents will typically increase and then peak near the end of the Adult stage. Requirements to attend children's soccer games, little league games, etc. may consequently progressively limit participation among Adults in 5K races and hence be associated with the slow decline in participation among females during this stage.

However, among the Masters group, increasing age can be accompanied by many factors that affect the frequency of competition or even the ability to complete a 5K in the requisite 60 plus minutes. Arthritis, heart disease, plantar fasciitis, tendonitis, joint replacements and many other ailments more common among older individuals may reduce performance. Some individuals may drop out of racing altogether because they do not wish to be among the last to finish or because they simply cannot safely complete a

5K at all. In addition, with age, injuries become more frequent and recovery times become longer so that both the ability to train and the availability for participation are more limited. Similarly, the youngest Children, may not yet be physically or emotionally able to safely complete a 5K within the required time frame.

If lower participation rates in the Child and Masters groups reflect a reduced ability to complete a 5K distance within the typical race cut-off time, then the performances recorded for these ages will show a bias for the more speedy individuals. On the other hand, we might anticipate very little bias in performances recorded for Adolescents and Adults since the (relatively) smaller variations in participation rates among these groups can be explained by something other than performance related factors.

As we will see, straggling rates tend to confirm our concern that performance related participation censoring can create a bias in the times recorded for older Masters and younger Children; i.e. the lower tails of these performance distributions will be disproportionately under represented. This begs the question as to how centiles should be adjusted in order to correct for bias introduced by performance related censoring of participation. For example, within the data collected here, there were 1857 males aged 66 and their median speed (929 of 1857) was 9.25 km/h (32 minutes and 26 seconds). However, the participation rate for 66 year old males was 11.42 per thousand population versus 40.93 per thousand for 42 year old males. Thus, with a standard participation rate of 40.93, the expected number of 66 year old runners would be 1857*40.93/11.42 = 6657. Consequently, the runner with a speed of 9.25 km/hr. is ranked (approximately) in the top 14% (929 of 6657), i.e. his Participation Corrected Centile (PCC) is about 86%. In essence, this individual out performed both the 928 slower participants plus the 4800 individuals who would be expected to participate but for their inability to safely complete the race in a timely manner.

4.2 Results: Stragglers

Age related straggling rates can be a proxy for the relative difficulty participants have completing a race, and hence give some insight into the relationship between changes in participation rates and changes in performance. Presumably a high number of individuals struggling to complete a race portends a correspondingly high number of individuals who are psychologically unwilling or physically unable to safely participate at all.

A "straggler" is here defined as individual whose performance falls among the bottom 2% of all participants in each race. However, individuals who finished at the same time as a straggling Child (within 20 seconds), were more than 5 years older than the child, and had the same last name as the child were considered "caretakers". Since only 83% of the Children had an easily recoverable name, the "caretaker" counts were proportionately adjusted. For each age, the number of "caretakers" was subtracted from the gross straggler counts.

By this definition, there were 20,136 stragglers and 702 caretakers. The average straggler speed was 5.08 km/hr. (3.16 mi/hr., corresponding to 59 minutes and 3 seconds). Figure 3 shows the actual and smoothed percent stragglers for Females and Males respectively. [Note: due to the relatively small number of participants at the highest ages, pooled estimates of straggling rates were used for 75 to 79, 80 to 84, and 85 to 89.]

Although the straggling rate for males is about half that of females, the overall patterns of the two genders are similar: a rapid decline during Childhood, a low and relatively stable straggling rate during Adolescence and Adulthood, followed by a large and continuous upturn starting a few years into the Masters life stage.

After ages 46 (males) and 41 (females) the straggling rate begins a continuous uptrend (Figure 3). The Masters upturn in straggling occurs slightly later than participation rates start their accelerating downturn in Figure 1. This is consistent with a lowered racing frequency, possibly due to injuries and slower healing, coming earlier than actual difficultly in completing a race. For Children, the turning points for participation rates and straggling rates appear to occur at about the same age.

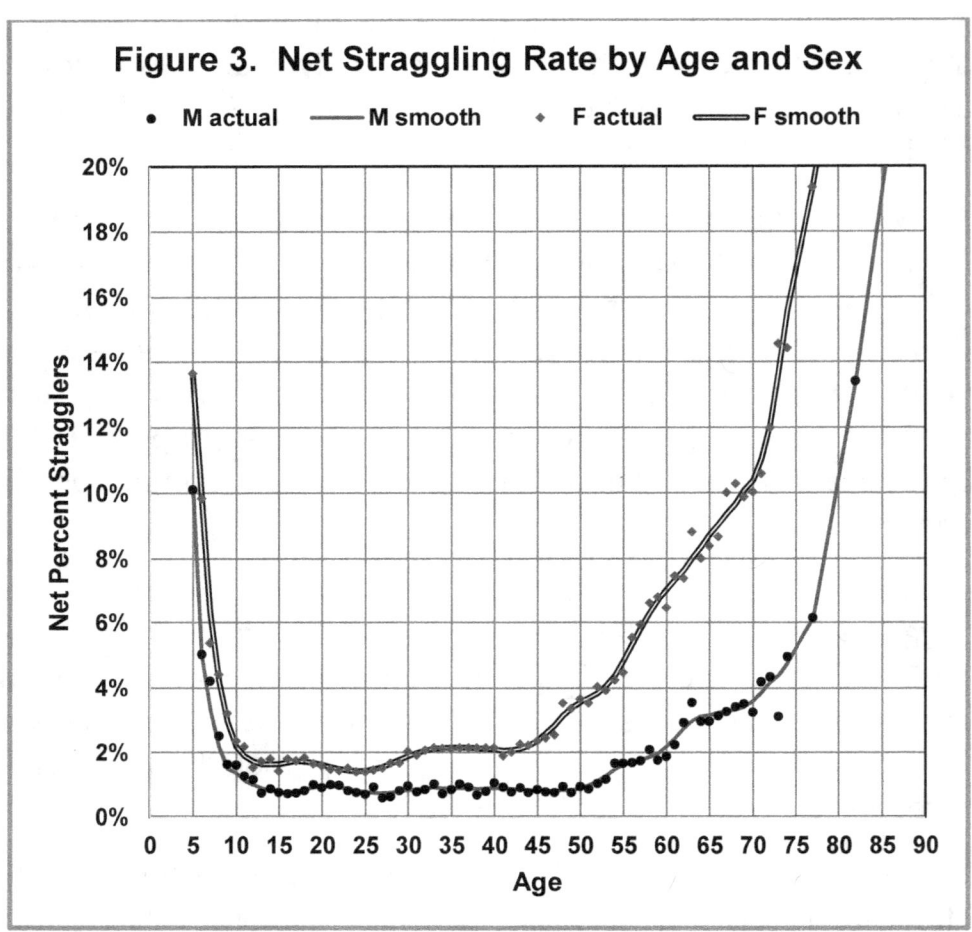

Figure 3. Net Straggling Rate by Age and Sex

4.3 Results: Correlation between Straggling and Participation Rates

In both the Child and Masters life stages and for both males and females there was a very strong negative correlation between the log of participation rates and the log of straggling rates. The correlation coefficients were as follows:

Male Children:	-0.987
Female Children:	-0.992
Male Masters:	-0.973
Female Masters:	-0.975

All of these correlations were highly statistically significant with $p<0.0001$ in each case. See Figures 4A and 4B.

On the other hand, none of the correlations between the log of participation rates and the log of straggling rates were statistically significant in the Adolescent and Adult life stages, $p>0.05$ in each case. Moreover, among both female and male Adolescents, the straggling rates did not differ significantly among the different ages, $p>0.05$ in both cases (chi squared with 12 df = 16.3 and 20.2, respectively).

The strong correlation between straggler and participation rates among Children and Masters is consistent with the assertion that changes in participation rates during these life stages largely correspond to performance changes affecting the ability and willingness to participate. However, the decline and then recovery in participation rates during Adolescence were not strongly associated with corresponding changes in straggling rates, supporting the earlier discussion that changes in participation rates during this life stage were primarily independent of performance ability.

Because of the disparate impact of participation rates across life states, Centiles for speed (or equivalently for time) will necessarily be corrected for participation rates in the Child and Masters Life stages, but not in the Adolescent and Adult stages. Consequently the results for the various life stages are discussed separately.

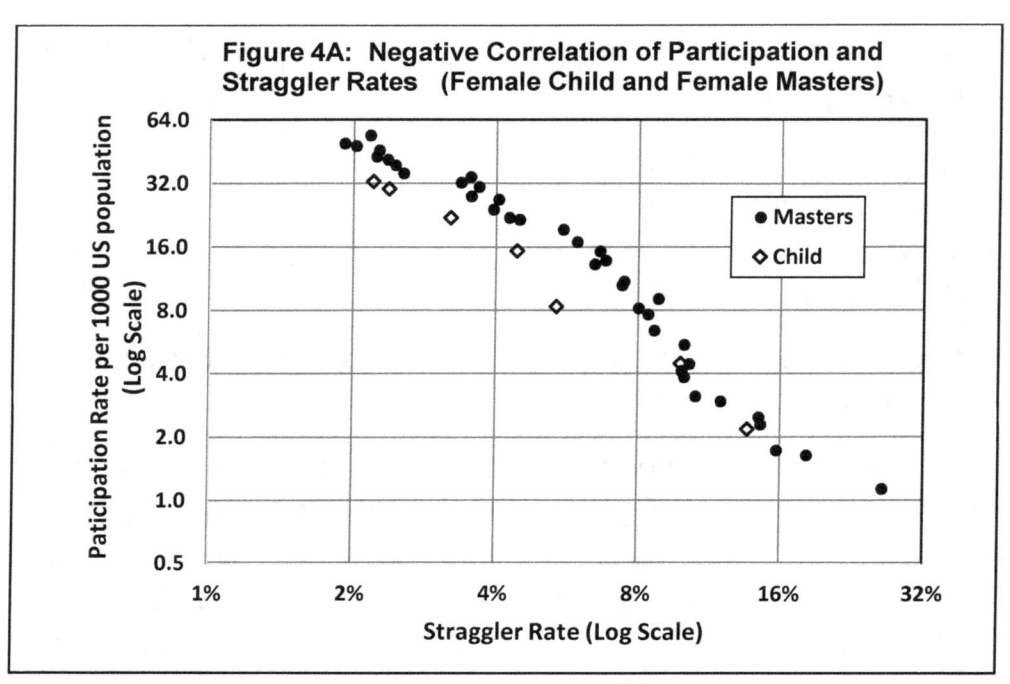

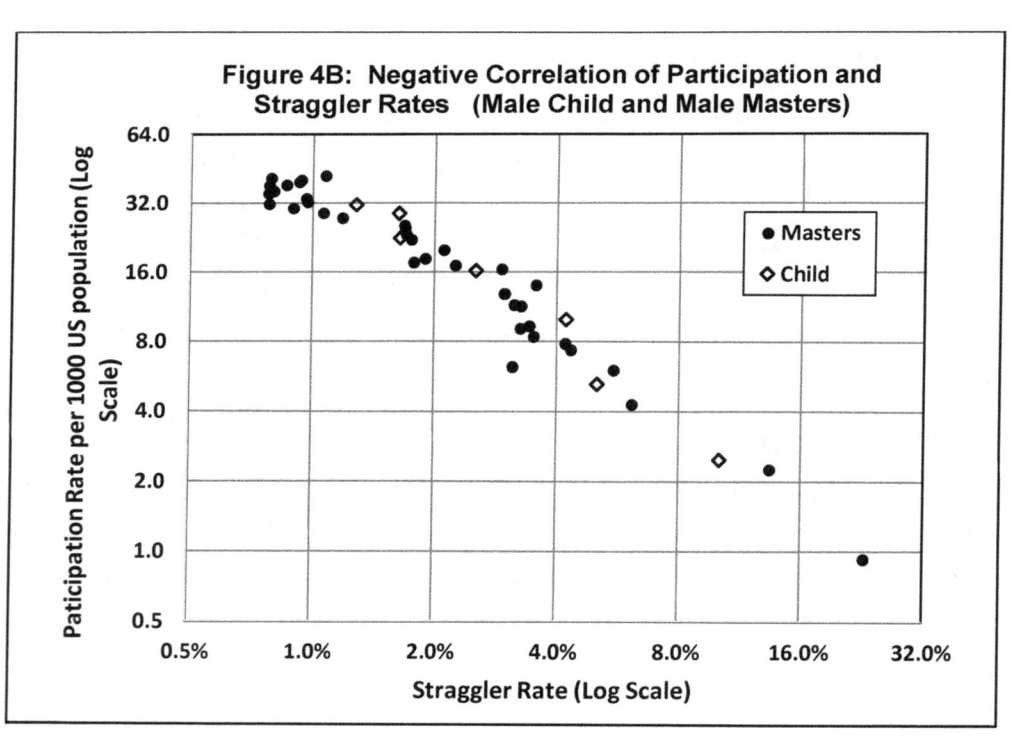

4.4 Results: Centiles for Speed, Adolescent and Adult Life Stages

Let's return to the earlier example of a father and son (ages 36 and 14) who both completed a 5K in 25 minutes. Based on the "WMA Age-grading calculator 2015" (www.howardgrubb.co.uk/athletics/), the father had an "Age-performance %" of 53.35%, but the son had an Age-performance % of 54.77%, so, using this metric, the son would be the clear winner on an age adjusted basis. In fact, the WMA calculator has the son with an age graded time 38 seconds faster than the father.

However, when we compare the father and son performances against their respective peer groups, we reach exactly the opposite conclusion! The son is faster than 55.3% of his same age peers whereas the father is faster than 69.6% of his peers. Among 36 year old males, the 55.3 centile corresponds to 26 minutes and 57 seconds indicating that, on this scale, the father is a minute and 57 seconds faster than the son.

The key to understanding this discrepancy is to recognize that the WMA standards are based on world record performances. For these to apply to "average" athletes, we must assume that average athletes and the super elite change at the same rate with age — and this is not the case. To illustrate, suppose another father and son pair are somewhat more elite in that they both complete the course in 17 minutes. In this case, the father is faster than 99.1% of his 36 year old peers and the son is faster than 99.8% of his 14 year old peer group. Thus, on a directional basis, the WMA calculator and the comparative peer group performances agree for these elite athletes even though they were diametrically opposed for average athletes.

Figure 5 shows the empirical probability density function (pdf) for the speeds of 14 and 36 year old males. The graph uses a one km/hr. wide moving average. Except for the tails, almost the entire distribution for 14 year olds is shifted approximately one km/h to the right of the distribution for 36 year olds; the medians of the 14 year old and 36 year old distributions are 11.63 and 10.78, respectively.

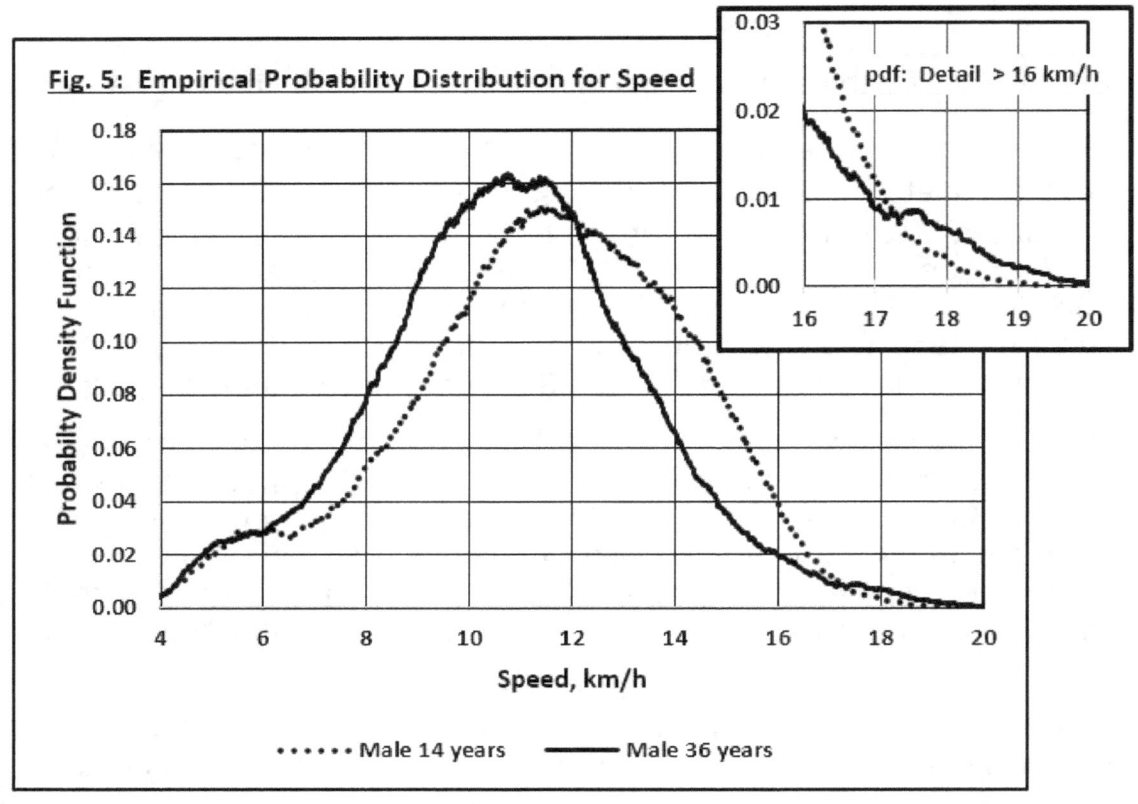

Fig. 5: Empirical Probability Distribution for Speed

However, as shown in the Figure 5 inset, the 36 year old pdf becomes dominant above about 17 km/hr. Thus, in comparison to 14 year olds, a higher percentage of 36 year olds exceed 17 km/hr.

4.5 Results: Age at Peak Performance

WMA uses "Age-grading factors" (positive numbers with values of 1 or less) to adjust performance based on age. For females, the factors are 1.0000 between ages 19 and 30, implying that no age adjustment is needed within this range. Participants older than 30 or younger than 19 have factors of less than 1. For example, the factor for a 39 year old female is 0.979, indicating, based on age alone, a 39 year old would be expected to be a about 2% slower than someone in the "ideal" 19-30 age range.

For any given performance centile, a similar set of age grading factors can be constructed by dividing the speed at each age by the maximum speed across all ages. For example, the maximum speed for the female 75th centile is 11.31 km/hour and it occurs at age 16. At age 39, the speed of the 75th centile is 10.29 km/hour, consequently with the 75th centile the age grading factor for a 39 year old female is 10.29/11.31 = 0.910.

Figure 6A compares the Female WMA Age-grading factors with age-grading factors generated by the Female 75th centile and by the 99.5th centile. The Savitzky-Golay smoothing filter was applied to the centile results shown in Figures 6A and 6B. The 75th and the 99.5th centiles show very different patterns from each other as well as from the WMA standards. Figure 6A graphically shows that a single set of age-grading factors cannot be applicable across a wide range of athletic abilities. Even though the 75th centile represents somewhat better than average runners, the peak performance for this group occurs before the WMA "sweet spot" (19-30 years) and several years before the peak in the 99.5th centile.

Table 1 shows how the age of peak performance differs among the various centiles. For both males and females the "average" participant (50th centile) peaks at age 17 whereas the truly superior runners (99.9th centile) peak at 25. However, as the centiles go from 50th to 99.9th the change in age at peak performance is much more abrupt for females and gradual for males.

At the other end of the female performance scale (10th – 30th centiles) the speeds suggest that the participants are walking or engaging in a mixture of running and walking (Minetti, et. al., 2003; Hreljac, et. al., 2002; Long, et. al., 2013). Walking at 7.7 km/hr. or 6.5 km/hr. (about 4.8 mph and 4 mph, respectively) are brisk speeds for walking a significant distance and may represent a good performance centile among walkers. In any case, Table 1 further illustrates the difficulty of using a single standard for age grading across a wide range of abilities.

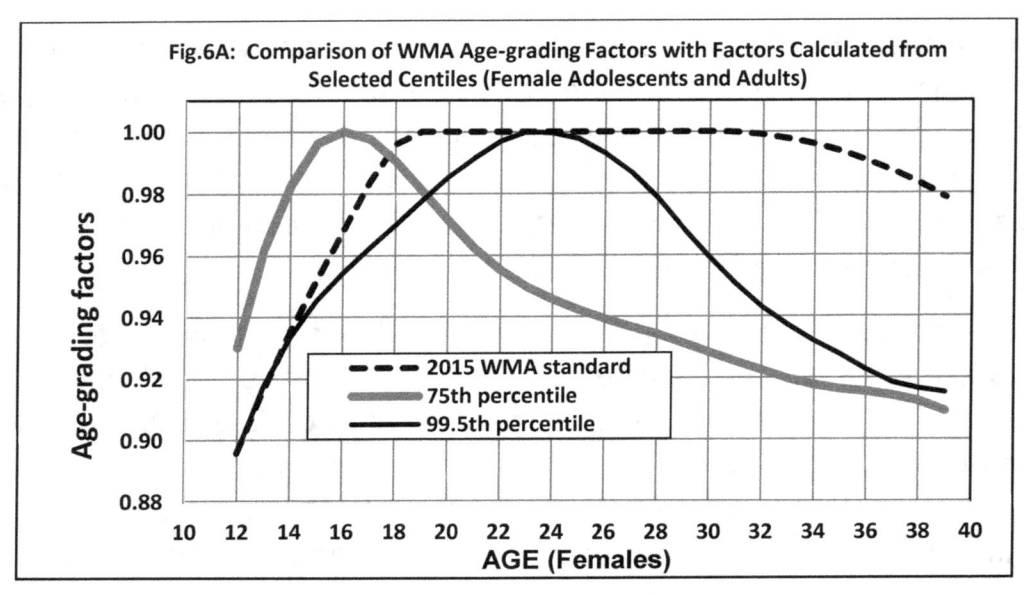

Fig.6A: Comparison of WMA Age-grading Factors with Factors Calculated from Selected Centiles (Female Adolescents and Adults)

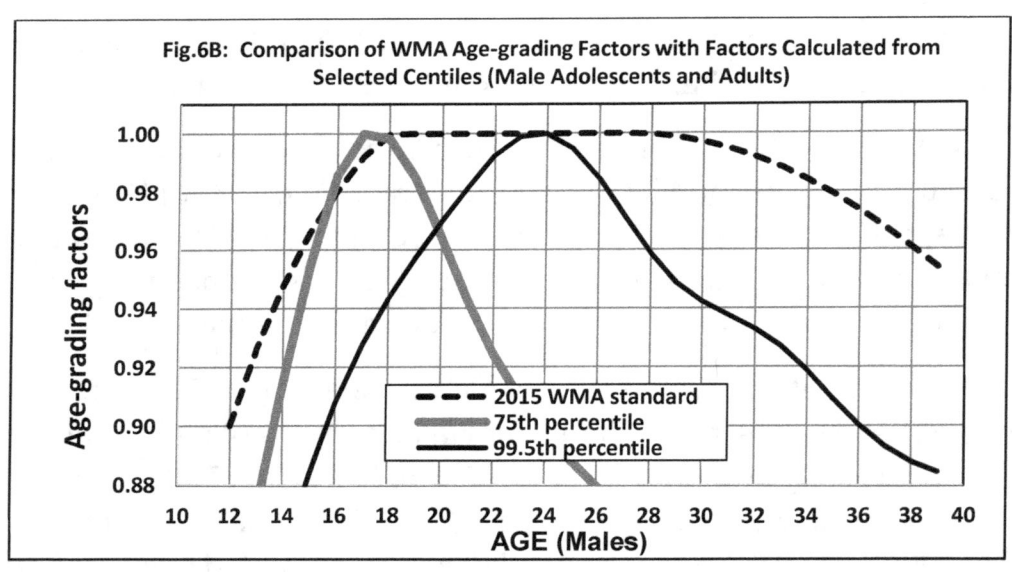

Fig.6B: Comparison of WMA Age-grading Factors with Factors Calculated from Selected Centiles (Male Adolescents and Adults)

Table 1: Age of Peak 5K Speed in Relation to Performance Centile

Centile	Age when Maximum Speed is Attained		Maximum Speed Attained (km/hr)		5K Time Elapsed at Peek Speed (mm:ss)	
	Female	Male	Female	Male	Female	Male
99.9%	25	25	17.9	21.4	16:44	14:02
99.5%	23	24	16.2	20.0	18:32	14:58
99%	22	23	15.4	19.4	19:27	15:26
98%	18	22	14.6	18.8	20:29	15:57
97%	17	21	14.2	18.3	21:04	16:22
96%	17	20	13.9	18.0	21:33	16:41
95%	17	20	13.7	17.7	21:57	16:57
94%	17	19	13.4	17.4	22:20	17:12
93%	16	19	13.2	17.2	22:40	17:24
92%	16	19	13.1	17.0	22:58	17:37
91%	16	19	12.9	16.8	23:15	17:51
90%	16	18	12.8	16.6	23:30	18:01
85%	16	18	12.2	15.9	24:37	18:51
80%	16	18	11.7	15.3	25:35	19:40
70%	16	17	11.0	14.2	27:22	21:07
60%	17	17	10.3	13.3	29:06	22:29
50%	17	17	9.7	12.5	30:49	23:57
40%	16	17	9.1	11.7	32:54	25:36
30%	21	17	8.5	10.9	35:27	27:28
20%	24	17	7.7	9.9	38:49	30:14
10%	25	17	6.5	8.3	46:02	36:13

4.6 Results: Simulation: Ages 12—39

In order to compare the different methods for identifying top performers within the Adolescent and Adult life stages, I ran 10,000 simulations for each of four different target race sizes: 50, 100, 200, and 600 participants. For each simulation, participants were randomly selected from the entire data set with probability equal to (target_race_size)/1,042,126. Within each simulated race approximately 24% of the participants were expected to be males 12—39 and 33% were expected to be females 12—39. The top male and female in each 12—39 age group was determined by 3 methods: (1) Unadjusted speed, i.e. the individual with the best time. (2) WMA age-grading and (3) the highest single year age centile. Only simulated races with an unequivocal highest centile were counted – i.e. no ties for first place.

Table 2: Comparison of using Unadjusted Speed vs WMA Age-Grading to identify Best Centile Performance between Ages 12 and 39.				
(Based on 10,000 simulated races for each race size)				
Overall Race Size (incl. males and females, all ages 5-89)	Gender	Avg. No. Participants between 12 and 39	Percent of simulations in which top performer was correctly identified	
			WMA age-grading	Unadjusted Speed
50	Females	17	81%	86%
	Males	12	79%	75%
100	Females	33	76%	83%
	Males	24	74%	69%
200	Females	66	75%	80%
	Males	47	71%	64%
600	Females	199	76%	77%
	Males	142	64%	55%

Table 2 shows the results of the simulation. Most noteworthy is that, for females, WMA age grading performed worse than simply using the unadjusted speed; i.e. the first individual to cross the finish line was more likely to have the highest centile than the individual with the best WMA age-grade. For males, the WMA age grade did perform better than unadjusted speed. However, it still did not correctly identify the top centile very well.

4.7 Participation Corrected Centiles, Masters Stage: Ages 40-89

"Fight, Fight, Fight!" shouted the ninetyish pre-race motivational speaker. "Fight for every breath, fight for every step, fight for every inch!" Clearly the race organizers on stage with this gentleman considered him to be a paragon of racing prowess when they selected him to speak to us prior to the annual Hannibal-Cannibal race. After the race, I came across this man and started questioning him. He was in the middle of explaining how he paced himself when he abruptly broke off our conversation to talk with a couple of young ladies who had obviously been paying attention to him. (They couldn't have been much over 75).

When I looked up earlier race results for this individual, I found that at 89 he had completed the 5K race in 44:40. The dataset collected here contained just 13 males 89 years old. Our motivational speaker had a better time than 10 of these individuals but was slower than three, so among same age participants he would be about the 75th centile. Now the 75th centile is somewhat above average, but in any race of more than 100 participants there will be dozens of individuals above the 75th centile and most would not be selected as exemplars of peak competitive performance. However, recognizing that only the smallest fraction of living 89 year olds are actually able and willing to safely complete a 5K suggests that we must account for participation rates in evaluating this individual's performance.

This raises the question: at what age should centiles be corrected for participation rates? The data here suggest that participation correction of the centiles begin at ages 41 (females) and 43 (males). These are the ages immediately following the accelerating decline in participation rates previously identified in figures 1, 2A and 2B. These ages also coincide with or immediately precede the upsurge in straggling rates seen in figure 3. Moreover, there are extremely strong correlations between participation rates and straggling rates starting at these ages (figures 4A and 4B). Consequently, participation rates for ages 40 (females) and 42 (males) are used as the basis for correcting all subsequent performance centiles.

Table 3: Compare Rankings based on Participation Corrected Centiles versus WMA Standards (Top 7 Male and Female Centiles; 294 total participants, Hannibal Cannibal 2005)

FEMALES

Gender	Age	Time	Speed km/hr.	Centile	Rank based on Centile	Rank based on WMA standards
F	47	20:32	14.61	99.7	1	1
F	18	20:11	14.86	98.5	2	3
F	14	21:14	14.13	97.9	3	2
F	18	21:16	14.11	96.7	4	4
F	56	28:01	10.71	96.6	5	11
F	69	44:21	6.76	96.6	6	101
F	53	26:46	11.21	96.2	7	8

MALES

Gender	Age	Time	Speed km/hr.	Centile	Rank based on Centile	Rank based on WMA standards
M	89	44:40	6.72	99.6	1	34
M	57	20:09	14.89	98.8	2	2
M	41	18:05	16.59	98.4	3	3
M	21	16:17	18.42	97.2	4	1
M	58	21:50	13.74	96.9	5	5
M	10	23:01	13.03	96.1	6	11
M	57	22:35	13.28	94.9	7	6

After correcting for participation rates, our 89 year old was in the 99.6[th] centile -- obviously more appropriate than his uncorrected centile. As Table 3 shows, the 89 year had the highest centile of any male in the race, and was second only to a 47 year old female who had a time of 20:32. (Who, although from out of the region, is an accomplished runner in her own right.) However, WMA age grading would have ranked him 34th among 141 males -- not very high at all. Similarly note that, based on centiles, the 6th ranked female would be ranked 101st using WMA age grading. Using world records plus the assumption that everyone ages at the same rate causes WMA age grading to substantially over estimate the capability of more typical older participants.

4.8 Participation Corrected Centiles for Speed, Child Stage

For both males and females during the child stage, participation rates climb rapidly with age and straggling rates decline rapidly. There is a very strong negative correlation of participation with straggling rates between the ages of 5 and 11.   By age 12 both males and females have reached very low straggling rates (1.2% and 1.7% respectively, Figure 3). As figures 2A and 2B show, the (locally) greatest deceleration in the childhood participation decline occurs at ages 12 (females) and 13 (males), suggesting participation adjustment should begin immediately preceding these ages. Since male and female participation rates are virtually identical between 8 and 15, the centiles for both genders are corrected for participation at ages 11 and below, using the participation at age 12 as a basis for correction.

5. Summary of Age Related Changes in Speed: 5 to 89

Figures 7A and 7B show the speeds of athletes in the 50th, 90th, 99th, and 99.9th participation corrected centiles (PCC). These speeds are corrected for participation rates in the Child and Masters stages and the curves are smoothed using the Savitzky-Golay filter as indicated earlier. Also shown are the speeds corresponding to the WMA age standards and the World Single Age Records--5 km Road from the Association of Road Racing Statisticians, http://www.arrs.net. (Note that the world road record for 82 year old males is below the 99.9th centile and considerably below records for nearby ages. Several results in the current dataset were also better than this record. Presumably, the record for 82 year old males could be eligible for an update at some point.)

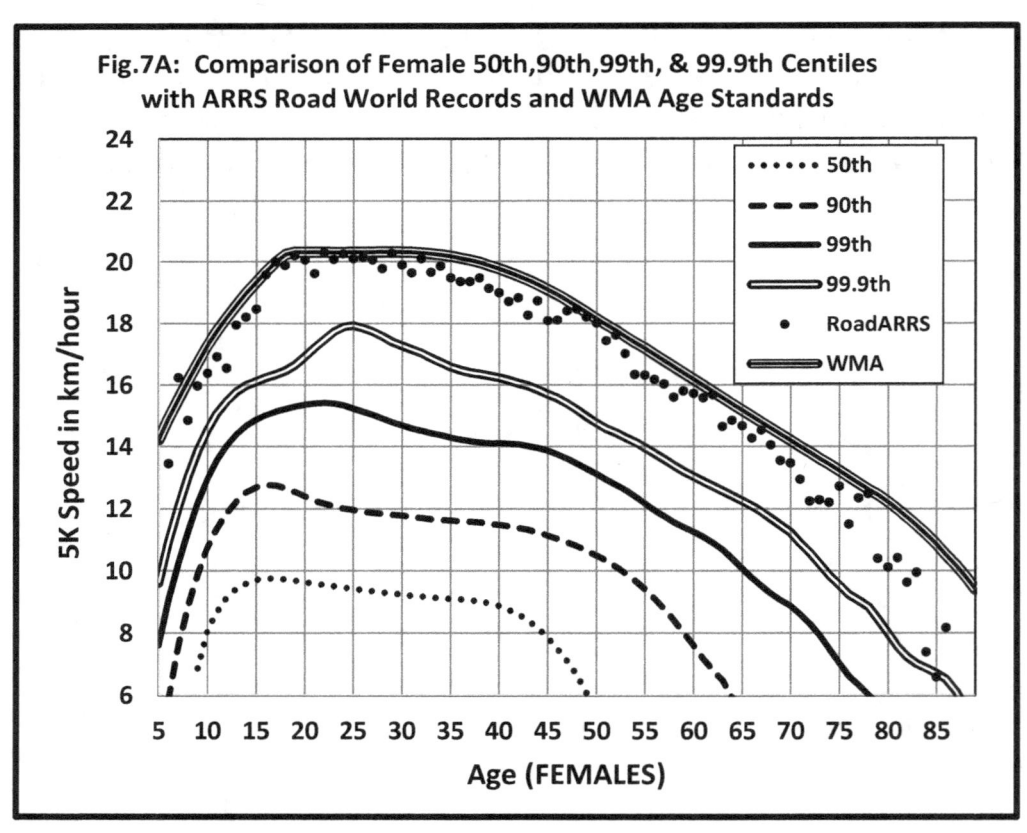

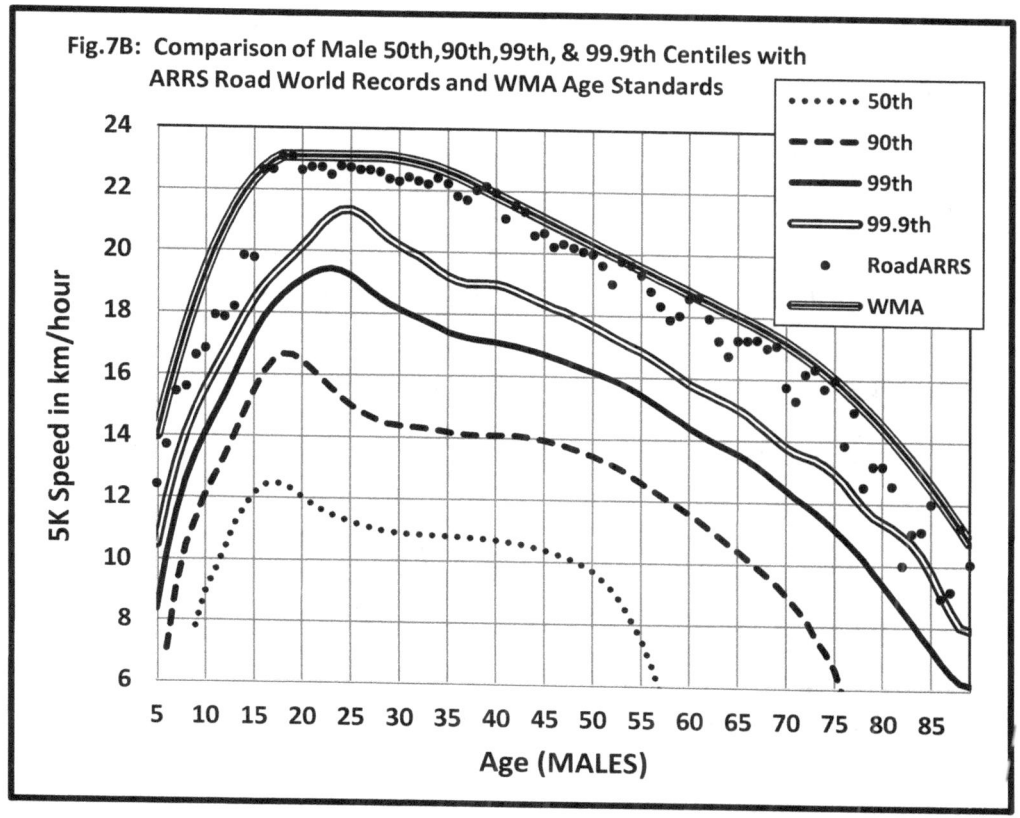

Fig.7B: Comparison of Male 50th,90th,99th, & 99.9th Centiles with ARRS Road World Records and WMA Age Standards

Although, as previously noted, there are differences among the various centiles in figures 7A and 7B, most do show a common pattern. In particular, and especially for males, after the age of peak performance, a period of rapid decline is followed by a plateauing in performance lasting several years. Subsequent to the years of plateau, speed again resumes an increasingly rapid decline. Each of the curves for the centiles has a section which is concave upward. This is not the case for the WMA standard for speed. The WMA curve is never concave upward (Jones, 2015).

Because these curves (Figures 7A & 7B) are not proportional to each other, bias is introduced when WMA standards are used to age grade performances of athletes who are less than world class.

Since all individuals achieving a given centile perform equivalently among their same age peers, a consistent approach to age-grading requires that the same age-graded time (or equivalently, age-graded speed) be assigned to each individual in a given centile. However, this is not the case with the current WMA age-grading process. For example, with 75 year old males, the 90th centile speed is 6.57 km/hr. Since the WMA "Factor" for 75 year old males is 0.6926, the WMA age-graded speed is 6.57/0.6926 = 9.49 km/hr. On the other hand, for 20 year olds, the WMA age graded speed for the 90th centile is 16.45 km/hr. Across all ages the median WMA age graded speed for the 90th centile is 14.63 km/hr. Consequently, the WMA age graded speed for a 75 year old in the 90th centile has a *negative* 35% bias while a 20 year old performing at the 90th centile has a *positive* 12% bias.

Figure 8 illustrates the percent bias across all ages for the 90th centile. Note that the very youngest and the oldest participants are put at a significant disadvantage, whereas, the Adolescent stage and the early Masters stage (between about 40 and 55 years) gain an inappropriate advantage from the current standards for WMA age-grading. Although the degree of bias and the exact age ranges vary somewhat, a similar pattern of bias follows for other centiles and for females: in every case the very youngest and oldest participants are unfairly disadvantaged.

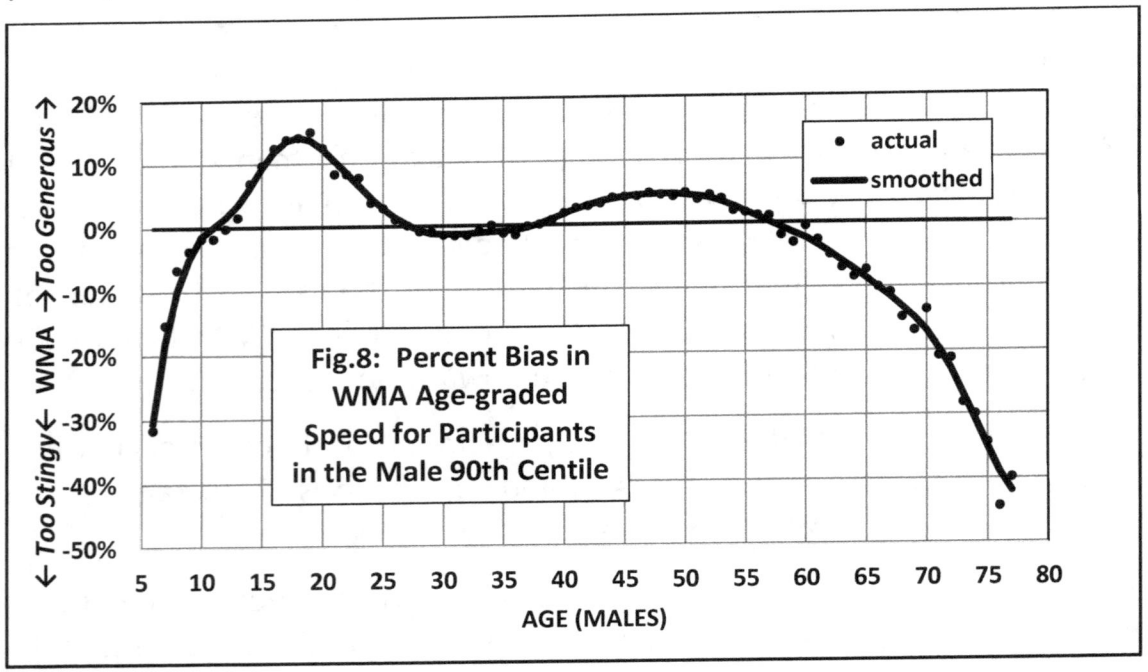

Fig.8: Percent Bias in WMA Age-graded Speed for Participants in the Male 90th Centile

6. Standards for Participation Corrected Centile Performance

Clearly age grading standards developed from the performances of the super elite are inappropriate for the average athlete or even for very good athletes who are not contenders for a world age record. Participation corrected centiles are a natural and easily understandable alternative. Although, no single standard can work for all levels of performance, Figures 7A and 7B suggest, and a more detailed look at the data confirm that nearby centiles are approximately parallel. Consequently, a <u>family</u> of smoothed centile standards works quite well. Using this approach, the standards were fitted for the following 27 centiles: 10th, 20th, 30th, 40th, 50th, 60th, 70th, 75th, 80th, 85th, 86th, 87th, 88th, 89th, 90th, 91st, 92nd, 93rd, 94th, 95th, 96th, 97th, 98th, 99th, 99.5th, 99.9th, and 99.95th. These centiles are concentrated more heavily on the upper end since this is where accuracy to the last decimal point is likely to be emphasized. As more data becomes available, it may be meaningful to include higher centiles; or even incorporate a smoothed version of world records at the upper end! For example, what centile corresponds to the "typical" world record?

For performances which do not lie precisely on one of the above standard centiles, probit interpolation can be used to calculate the relevant centile. This is the method used to construct an excel spreadsheet which generated the centiles shown in table 3. However, in most situations ordinary linear interpolation is sufficiently accurate without the need to resort to probit interpolation.

[Example of probit interpolation for the third ranked male, age 41, in table 3, who had a speed of 16.59 km/hr.: The standard speed corresponding to the 98th centile for 41 year old males is 16.33 km/hr. and for the 99th centile it is 17.03 km/hr. Using the inverse standard normal distribution shows the probits for the 98th and 99th centiles are 2.0537 and 2.3263 standard deviations, respectively. Interpolating gives the probit corresponding to a speed of 16.59 km/hr. as 2.1541 standard deviations. For the cumulative normal distribution, 2.1541 standard deviations corresponds to a probability of 0.9844. Consequently, with probit interpolation, this individual is at the 98.44th centile. However, note that ordinary interpolation calculates the centile for this individual as the 98.37th — probably close enough for most applications.]

Discussion

Someone familiar with current age grading standards based on world records may be stunned to discover the large differences with standards developed from actual 5K races. Certainly the 18 year old male with a time of 16 minutes might be surprised to learn his performance is no more exceptional than that of a 74 year old woman who completes the course in just 40 minutes. But, of course, he should be proud of his grandmother, and consider that perhaps he inherited some of his drive and determination from her.

Given the bias and the other issues with the current WMA approach to age grading, the question naturally arises as to why hasn't this been replaced by centiles or some other more appropriate methodology? Several reasons present themselves, not the least of which is just the glamor associated with comparing oneself to world class runners. Figure 8 suggests a more Machiavellian explanation. Many of the more serious runners become interested in age grading after about 40 years of age. During the years immediately following, the bias of the current WMA approach becomes progressively larger and consequently these runners will be more prone to support a methodology that makes them look unusually good. (Of course their enthusiasm may be dashed about 20 years later when the bias starts to become negative.)

However, possibly the most significant reason centiles have not come into widespread use is the lack of an appropriate methodology for dealing with both participation censoring and with the great variability in population sizes among the ages. The approach presented here addresses these two methodological issues.

One unfortunate by-product of excessive focus on world records at the expense of studying the full spectrum of abilities is that insights into the entire population are likely to be missed. One curious example of this is the suggestion that laws and economic policies relating to aging should be revisited because 85 year old world and U.S. record holders can run quite well (Fair, 1994). In fact among these elites, an 85 year old man runs two-thirds as fast as a 55 year old record holder. However, as the data here suggest, the fraction of 85 year old men who are even willing and able to complete a 5K is less than 5% of what it was when they were 55.

One quite interesting feature of the data is that the probability distribution of speeds for each age does not fit a normal distribution. A composite of three distributions is required to give a good fit. This pattern is consistent across a wide range of ages. One of these distributions clearly identifies the walkers and the other two distributions split the runners into two distinct subgroups at each age. This raises many questions for future research. How do individuals change between the two running groups as they age? Is there a distinctive gait that differentiates the two groups? Can world record holders be reasonably classified as belonging to the top end of the faster running group or must they be considered to be drawn from an entirely different fourth subpopulation?

Another question is whether other distances (10K, half marathon, etc.) follow the same patterns as were observed for the 5K. With increasingly ubiquitous electronic race timing and the employment of professional electronic timing services in all but the smallest races, there is much data available for determining participation corrected centiles for races of all the popular distances.

Certainly a consortium of several regional timing services would have sufficient data to maintain very accurate standards for participation corrected centiles in all of the popular distances. Recognizing that their data played a significant role in developing the standards might even encourage more timing services to offer age grading services. And more accurate and more understandable age grading methodology might encourage more participation, better training, and consequently higher speeds among race participants. But then of course, we might have to update the standards.

7. Tables of 5K Times for Participation Corrected Centiles

The times required to achieve selected participation corrected centiles are shown in Tables 4i-4vi (females) and 5i-5vi (males). I have converted the speeds into times, since this will be more familiar to most people. For example, using Table 4iv, a 40 year old female with a time of 25 minutes is between the 93rd and 94th centile. Interpolation can be used if a more precise centile estimate is required. Since many races have a cut-off time only a little above an hour, these tables are not applicable for times over 60 minutes. Several cells show "<60" indicating the minimum centile assigned to anyone of the applicable age completing the race in less than 60 minutes. For example, a 71 year old male (Table 5vi) with a time of 50 minutes falls between the 80th and 85th centiles.

Table 4i   Child
Time (in Minutes:Seconds) for Selected Centiles

AGE ↓	↙ FEMALE Centile ↘											
	30th	40th	50th	60th	70th	75th	80th	85th	86th	87th	88th	89th
5	---	---	---	---	---	---	---	---	---	---	---	---
6	---	---	---	---	---	---	---	---	---	<60	57:31	54:42
7	---	---	---	---	---	<60	50:21	44:17	43:20	44:59	42:57	41:49
8	---	---	<60	51:23	43:51	44:41	40:01	37:01	36:29	36:06	35:26	34:53
9	<60	51:04	44:22	41:35	37:30	36:05	34:13	32:31	32:11	31:16	31:04	30:45
10	44:02	42:34	38:42	36:03	33:31	31:32	30:43	29:36	29:21	28:45	28:35	28:19
11	40:38	37:43	35:09	32:46	30:56	29:27	28:44	27:46	27:33	27:15	27:01	26:45

AGE ↓	↙ FEMALE Centile ↘											
	90th	91st	92nd	93rd	94th	95th	96th	97th	98th	99th	99.5th	99.9th
5	---	---	---	---	<60	57:44	52:24	48:53	44:23	39:15	35:48	31:13
6	52:20	49:50	47:41	45:49	45:29	43:08	40:53	38:51	36:18	33:18	31:04	27:29
7	40:43	39:37	38:36	37:37	36:35	35:27	34:19	32:58	31:19	29:21	27:47	24:52
8	34:16	33:44	33:10	32:34	31:30	30:51	30:12	29:12	28:02	26:36	25:24	22:59
9	30:21	30:02	29:40	29:15	28:33	28:03	27:33	26:47	25:50	24:38	23:38	21:37
10	28:00	27:43	27:25	27:04	26:36	26:10	25:43	25:06	24:17	23:13	22:19	20:37
11	26:28	26:11	25:54	25:35	25:10	24:46	24:21	23:49	23:07	22:09	21:22	19:54

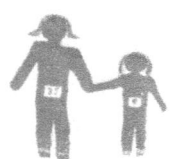

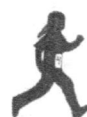

FEMALE Ages 12-24   **FEMALE Ages 12-24**

Table 4ii Adolescent
Time (in Minutes:Seconds) for Selected Centiles

AGE ↓	FEMALE Centile ↙ ↘											
	30th	40th	50th	60th	70th	75th	80th	85th	86th	87th	88th	89th
12	38:19	34:54	32:55	31:04	29:23	28:24	27:31	26:32	26:19	26:03	25:49	25:34
13	36:49	33:44	31:49	30:10	28:27	27:30	26:37	25:39	25:27	25:14	25:00	24:46
14	36:08	33:20	31:18	29:35	27:51	26:57	26:03	25:05	24:52	24:41	24:26	24:13
15	35:48	32:59	30:56	29:12	27:29	26:40	25:43	24:45	24:33	24:20	24:06	23:53
16	35:40	32:54	30:49	29:06	27:22	26:31	25:35	24:37	24:25	24:12	23:58	23:45
17	35:35	32:54	30:49	29:06	27:25	26:35	25:39	24:40	24:28	24:14	24:00	23:47
18	35:33	32:55	30:52	29:12	27:35	26:46	25:50	24:51	24:39	24:25	24:10	23:57
19	35:29	32:57	30:59	29:22	27:49	27:01	26:06	25:07	24:55	24:41	24:25	24:11
20	35:27	33:01	31:08	29:34	28:04	27:18	26:23	25:23	25:11	24:58	24:42	24:27
21	35:27	33:06	31:18	29:47	28:20	27:33	26:39	25:40	25:27	25:14	24:58	24:43
22	35:27	33:11	31:27	29:59	28:33	27:46	26:52	25:53	25:41	25:27	25:12	24:56
23	35:28	33:17	31:36	30:08	28:42	27:55	27:03	26:05	25:52	25:38	25:23	25.07
24	35:33	33:25	31:44	30:16	28:49	28:02	27:11	26:13	26:00	25:47	25:31	25:16

AGE ↓	FEMALE Centile ↙ ↘											
	90th	91st	92nd	93rd	94th	95th	96th	97th	98th	99th	99.5th	99.9th
12	25:19	25:03	24:45	24:26	24:07	23:44	23:21	22:52	22:16	21:23	20:41	19:23
13	24:31	24:15	23:58	23:39	23:21	23:00	22:37	22:10	21:38	20:50	20:12	19:01
14	23:58	23:43	23:26	23:07	22:49	22:28	22:06	21:40	21:11	20:26	19:51	18:46
15	23:38	23:23	23:06	22:48	22:29	22:09	21:46	21:21	20:53	20:10	19:36	18:37
16	23:30	23:15	22:58	22:40	22:20	21:59	21:36	21:09	20:41	19:58	19:25	18:30
17	23:31	23:16	22:59	22:40	22:20	21:57	21:33	21:04	20:33	19:49	19:15	18:23
18	23:41	23:26	23:07	22:48	22:26	22:02	21:36	21:05	20:29	19:42	19:06	18:14
19	23:55	23:41	23:21	23:02	22:39	22:12	21:45	21:09	20:29	19:36	18:57	18:02
20	24:12	23:57	23:37	23:17	22:53	22:25	21:56	21:17	20:33	19:31	18:48	17:46
21	24:27	24:12	23:53	23:32	23:08	22:39	22:08	21:27	20:40	19:29	18.41	17:28
22	24:40	24:25	24:06	23:45	23:21	22:52	22:21	21:38	20:47	19:27	18:35	17:11
23	24:51	24:36	24:17	23:57	23:33	23:04	22:33	21:49	20:55	19:29	13:32	16:56
24	24:59	24:44	24:26	24:06	23:42	23:15	22:44	22:01	21:04	19:34	18:32	16:47

Table 4iii   Adult
Time (in Minutes:Seconds) for Selected Centiles

AGE ↓	30th	40th	50th	60th	70th	75th	80th	85th	86th	87th	88th	89th
25	35:40	33:33	31:52	30:23	28:56	28:08	27:18	26:20	26:07	25:54	25:38	25:24
26	35:49	33:42	32:00	30:29	29:01	28:14	27:24	26:25	26:12	25:59	25:44	25:30
27	36:01	33:51	32:08	30:35	29:06	28:18	27:29	26:30	26:17	26:04	25:50	25:35
28	36:13	34:01	32:15	30:41	29:11	28:23	27:33	26:34	26:21	26:08	25:54	25:39
29	36:26	34:10	32:23	30:47	29:17	28:28	27:38	26:38	26:25	26:12	25:58	25:43
30	36:39	34:19	32:30	30:54	29:23	28:34	27:43	26:43	26:30	26:17	26:02	25:47
31	36:50	34:27	32:36	31:00	29:28	28:40	27:48	26:48	26:35	26:21	26:07	25:51
32	36:59	34:34	32:42	31:06	29:33	28:45	27:53	26:53	26:40	26:26	26:11	25:55
33	37:10	34:43	32:49	31:12	29:38	28:50	27:57	26:58	26:45	26:31	26:16	26:00
34	37:18	34:50	32:55	31:17	29:42	28:54	28:01	27:02	26:48	26:35	26:19	26:04
35	37:24	34:56	33:00	31:20	29:45	28:56	28:03	27:05	26:51	26:37	26:22	26:07
36	37:29	35:01	33:04	31:22	29:46	28:58	28:05	27:06	26:53	26:39	26:24	26:10
37	37:36	35:07	33:09	31:26	29:49	29:00	28:07	27:08	26:55	26:41	26:26	26:12
38	37:50	35:17	33:16	31:31	29:53	29:04	28:10	27:11	26:58	26:44	26:29	26:14
39	38:18	35:34	33:29	31:41	30:00	29:10	28:16	27:15	27:02	26:49	26:33	26:18

AGE ↓	90th	91st	92nd	93rd	94th	95th	96th	97th	98th	99th	99.5th	99.9th
25	25:06	24:50	24:33	24:13	23:49	23:24	22:52	22:10	21:13	19:40	18:34	16:44
26	25:12	24:56	24:38	24:18	23:54	23:30	22:59	22:18	21:22	19:48	18:40	16:49
27	25:17	25:00	24:42	24:22	23:59	23:35	23:03	22:24	21:29	19:57	18:47	16:56
28	25:21	25:04	24:45	24:25	24:02	23:38	23:07	22:28	21:36	20:06	18:56	17:06
29	25:25	25:07	24:48	24:27	24:05	23:41	23:10	22:33	21:44	20:16	19:08	17:16
30	25:29	25:11	24:51	24:31	24:09	23:44	23:14	22:37	21:50	20:25	19:19	17:23
31	25:33	25:15	24:56	24:35	24:13	23:47	23:18	22:42	21:54	20:32	19:29	17:30
32	25:38	25:20	25:01	24:39	24:18	23:51	23:22	22:46	21:58	20:40	19:39	17:38
33	25:43	25:25	25:06	24:44	24:22	23:56	23:26	22:49	22:02	20:46	19:46	17:47
34	25:47	25:30	25:10	24:48	24:26	23:59	23:30	22:52	22:06	20:53	19:53	17:57
35	25:50	25:32	25:14	24:52	24:29	24:03	23:33	22:56	22:10	20:58	19:59	18:06
36	25:53	25:35	25:16	24:54	24:32	24:06	23:36	23:00	22:14	21:04	20:05	18:13
37	25:55	25:37	25:18	24:57	24:34	24:10	23:40	23:05	22:19	21:09	20:10	18:19
38	25:58	25:40	25:21	25:00	24:37	24:14	23:45	23:10	22:24	21:13	20:13	18:21
39	26:02	25:44	25:25	25:04	24:41	24:18	23:49	23:15	22:27	21:15	20:15	18:24

FEMALE Ages 40-54 **FEMALE Ages 40-54**

Table 4iv   Early Masters
Time (in Minutes:Seconds) for Selected Centiles

AGE ↓	↙ FEMALE Centile ↘											
	30th	40th	50th	60th	70th	75th	80th	85th	86th	87th	88th	89th
40	39:07	36:02	33:48	31:56	30:11	29:18	28:23	27:21	27:08	26:55	26:39	26:23
41	40:39	36:48	34:16	32:17	30:26	29:31	28:33	27:30	27:17	27:03	26:47	26:30
42	42:41	37:50	34:52	32:41	30:43	29:45	28:45	27:40	27:27	27:12	26:56	26:39
43	45:33	39:10	35:41	33:11	31:03	30:02	28:59	27:52	27:38	27:22	27:06	26:49
44	49:08	41:08	36:44	33:46	31:26	30:20	29:15	28:06	27:51	27:34	27:18	27:00
45	53:50	43:40	38:05	34:28	31:52	30:42	29:33	28:21	28:06	27:49	27:32	27:13
46	<60	47:12	39:59	35:25	32:24	31:08	29:54	28:39	28:23	28:06	27:48	27:29
47	<60	52:04	42:10	36:33	33:03	31:38	30:19	29:00	28:43	28:25	28:07	27:48
48	<60	58:59	45:08	38:15	33:52	32:16	30:48	29:24	29:06	28:47	28:28	28:08
49	---	<60	49:04	40:23	34:58	33:03	31:24	29:52	29:33	29:13	28:53	28:32
50	---	<60	54:21	42:45	36:16	34:02	32:06	30:23	30:02	29:41	29:20	28:58
51	---	---	<60	46:00	38:15	35:14	32:55	30:58	30:36	30:14	29:51	29:28
52	---	---	<60	50:25	40:25	36:42	33:53	31:39	31:15	30:51	30:27	30:01
53	---	---	<60	56:28	42:48	38:25	35:12	32:31	32:04	31:37	31:11	30:42
54	---	---	---	<60	45:52	40:45	36:46	33:36	33:04	32:33	32:02	31:30

AGE ↓	↙ FEMALE Centile ↘											
	90th	91st	92nd	93rd	94th	95th	96th	97th	98th	99th	99.5th	99.9th
40	26:07	25:49	25:30	25:09	24:46	24:22	23:54	23:18	22:29	21:16	20:15	18:29
41	26:14	25:57	25:37	25:16	24:52	24:28	23:59	23:22	22:32	21:18	20:15	18:35
42	26:23	26:04	25:44	25:23	24:59	24:33	24:03	23:25	22:35	21:20	20:16	18:41
43	26:32	26:13	25:53	25:32	25:06	24:40	24:08	23:30	22:39	21:24	20:20	18:48
44	26:43	26:24	26:03	25:41	25:15	24:47	24:15	23:37	22:45	21:29	20:28	18:56
45	26:55	26:36	26:15	25:52	25:25	24:57	24:24	23:45	22:53	21:37	20:38	19:05
46	27:11	26:51	26:29	26:05	25:38	25:09	24:35	23:57	23:05	21:48	20:50	19:15
47	27:28	27:07	26:46	26:21	25:54	25:23	24:50	24:11	23:19	22:02	21:06	19:29
48	27:48	27:26	27:04	26:38	26:11	25:39	25:06	24:27	23:35	22:18	21:22	19:45
49	28:11	27:48	27:25	26:59	26:32	25:59	25:25	24:45	23:54	22:34	21:40	20:02
50	28:36	28:13	27:49	27:21	26:54	26:20	25:45	25:04	24:14	22:52	21:56	20:18
51	29:04	28:39	28:14	27:45	27:17	26:43	26:07	25:25	24:33	23:10	22:12	20:33
52	29:36	29:10	28:43	28:13	27:43	27:08	26:30	25:46	24:52	23:29	22:27	20:46
53	30:15	29:46	29:17	28:46	28:14	27:37	26:56	26:11	25:13	23:49	22:43	20:59
54	31:00	30:28	29:57	29:23	28:48	28:08	27:25	26:38	25:37	24:12	23:01	21:11

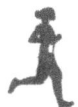

Table 4v   Middle Masters
Time (in Minutes:Seconds) for Selected Centiles

AGE ↓	↙ FEMALE Centile ↘											
	30th	40th	50th	60th	70th	75th	80th	85th	86th	87th	88th	89th
55	---	---	---	<60	49:46	43:28	38:51	34:57	34:18	33:41	33:04	32:27
56	---	---	---	<60	54:49	47:04	41:44	36:43	35:53	35:06	34:21	33:36
57	---	---	---	---	<60	51:51	44:27	38:47	37:52	36:51	35:55	35:02
58	---	---	---	---	<60	58:20	48:06	41:27	40:11	38:59	37:50	36:43
59	---	---	---	---	---	<60	52:49	44:18	42:43	41:19	39:58	38:40
60	---	---	---	---	---	<60	59:00	47:06	45:37	44:05	42:30	41:00
61	---	---	---	---	---	---	<60	50:39	48:40	47:13	45:30	43:45
62	---	---	---	---	---	---	<60	55:37	52:12	50:34	48:39	46:26
63	---	---	---	---	---	---	---	<60	57:11	54:09	51:51	49:33
64	---	---	---	---	---	---	---	---	<60	58:03	55:09	53:02
65	---	---	---	---	---	---	---	---	---	<60	58:31	56:57
66	---	---	---	---	---	---	---	---	---	---	---	---
67	---	---	---	---	---	---	---	---	---	---	---	---
68	---	---	---	---	---	---	---	---	---	---	---	---
69	---	---	---	---	---	---	---	---	---	---	---	---

AGE ↓	↙ FEMALE Centile ↘											
	90th	91st	92nd	93rd	94th	95th	96th	97th	98th	99th	99.5th	99.9th
55	31:52	31:17	30:42	30:04	29:26	28:43	27:57	27:08	26:03	24:38	23:22	21:27
56	32:55	32:15	31:33	30:52	30:09	29:21	28:33	27:42	26:33	25:04	23:45	21:44
57	34:10	33:24	32:34	31:46	30:57	30:04	29:13	28:19	27:05	25:31	24:10	22:04
58	35:39	34:42	33:41	32:44	31:49	30:50	29:54	28:55	27:36	25:56	24:34	22:24
59	37:25	36:11	34:57	33:50	32:46	31:39	30:36	29:30	28:04	26:19	24:56	22:43
60	39:20	37:51	36:27	35:07	33:52	32:34	31:21	30:05	28:31	26:40	25:15	22:59
61	41:42	39:54	38:11	36:37	35:09	33:38	32:10	30:43	29:01	27:04	25:36	23:17
62	44:07	42:08	40:08	38:21	36:36	34:51	33:08	31:28	29:36	27:31	25:59	23:33
63	46:19	44:38	42:24	40:27	38:24	36:22	34:20	32:28	30:22	28:08	26:28	23:53
64	49:18	47:36	44:38	42:42	40:25	38:14	35:54	33:47	31:23	28:54	27:02	24:10
65	54:19	51:04	47:34	45:33	43:00	40:26	37:47	35:24	32:36	29:46	27:40	24:29
66	<60	55:10	51:56	49:00	46:08	43:10	39:52	37:09	33:53	30:41	28:21	24:49
67	---	<60	58:07	53:02	49:37	45:43	42:13	39:05	35:12	31:35	29:01	25:13
68	---	---	<60	57:35	52:53	48:47	44:50	41:03	36:30	32:24	29:36	25:40
69	---	---	---	<60	56:04	51:49	47:00	42:37	37:46	33:07	30:04	26:12

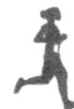

FEMALE Ages 70-89   **FEMALE Ages 70-89**

Table 4vi   Later Masters
Time (in Minutes:Seconds) for Selected Centiles

AGE ↓	↙ FEMALE Centile ↘											
	90th	91st	92nd	93rd	94th	95th	96th	97th	98th	99th	99.5th	99.9th
70	---	---	---	<60	59:02	55:08	50:40	44:48	38:59	33:49	30:29	26:43
71	---	---	---	---	<60	58:43	54:09	46:24	40:39	34:52	31:09	27:33
72	---	---	---	---	---	<60	57:26	48:11	42:41	36:08	32:01	28:24
73	---	---	---	---	---	---	<60	51:02	44:45	37:52	33:16	29:25
74	---	---	---	---	---	---	<60	57:13	48:50	40:04	35:03	30:27
75	---	---	---	---	---	---	---	<60	53:06	42:35	37:10	31:27
76	---	---	---	---	---	---	---	<60	56:43	45:20	39:39	32:26
77	---	---	---	---	---	---	---	<60	59:55	47:29	41:55	33:13
78	---	---	---	---	---	---	---	---	<60	49:48	43:46	33:57
79	---	---	---	---	---	---	---	---	<60	52:19	45:57	35:35
80	---	---	---	---	---	---	---	---	<60	54:24	46:47	37:25
81	---	---	---	---	---	---	---	---	<60	56:33	47:59	39:38
82	---	---	---	---	---	---	---	---	<60	58:35	50:21	41:33
83	---	---	---	---	---	---	---	---	---	<60	53:05	42:53
84	---	---	---	---	---	---	---	---	---	<60	57:01	43:42
85	---	---	---	---	---	---	---	---	---	---	<60	44:42
86	---	---	---	---	---	---	---	---	---	---	<60	45:50
87	---	---	---	---	---	---	---	---	---	---	<60	48:33
88	---	---	---	---	---	---	---	---	---	---	<60	52:38
89	---	---	---	---	---	---	---	---	---	---	<60	58:45

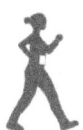

Table 5i   Child
Time (in Minutes:Seconds) for Selected Centiles

AGE ↓	↙ MALE Centile ↘											
	30th	40th	50th	60th	70th	75th	80th	85th	86th	87th	88th	89th
5	---	---	---	---	---	---	---	---	---	---	---	---
6	---	---	---	---	---	---	<60	58:34	53:57	50:46	48:28	46:22
7	---	---	---	---	<60	47:30	40:46	40:06	38:45	37:38	36:43	35:48
8	---	---	<60	43:22	36:44	36:54	33:57	31:58	31:31	31:03	30:36	30:08
9	<60	45:42	38:26	36:05	32:28	31:09	29:43	27:40	27:32	27:19	27:03	26:47
10	40:08	37:56	34:02	31:34	29:25	27:45	26:58	25:44	25:38	25:28	25:15	25:02
11	35:56	33:13	30:54	28:37	27:09	26:00	25:21	24:31	24:22	24:12	23:59	23:48

AGE ↓	↙ MALE Centile ↘											
	90th	91st	92nd	93rd	94th	95th	96th	97th	98th	99th	99.5th	99.9th
5	---	---	---	<60	55:30	50:45	47:11	43:31	40:04	35:28	32:01	28:34
6	44:05	42:22	40:38	41:20	39:15	37:27	35:52	34:09	32:18	29:48	27:57	25:13
7	34:50	34:02	33:11	32:20	31:36	30:45	29:52	28:55	27:45	26:14	25:09	22:54
8	29:39	29:14	28:45	27:40	27:23	26:55	26:20	25:43	24:54	23:52	23:08	21:16
9	26:31	26:15	25:57	25:27	25:14	24:52	24:25	23:55	23:15	22:25	21:46	20:11
10	24:50	24:36	24:22	24:02	23:49	23:28	23:05	22:38	22:03	21:19	20:40	19:20
11	23:36	23:23	23:10	22:53	22:40	22:21	22:00	21:35	21:04	20:24	19:46	18:37

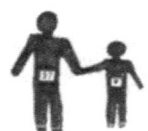

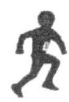

MALE Ages 12-24   **MALE Ages 12-24**

Table 5ii   Adolescent
Time (in Minutes:Seconds) for Selected Centiles

AGE ↓	MALE Centile ↙ ↘											
	30th	40th	50th	60th	70th	75th	80th	85th	86th	87th	88th	89th
12	32:58	30:12	28:37	26:48	25:30	24:45	24:05	23:20	23:11	23:01	22:50	22:40
13	30:50	28:22	26:55	25:29	24:10	23:28	22:51	22:09	22:01	21:51	21:41	21:32
14	29:17	27:16	25:44	24:18	22:59	22:19	21:42	21:03	20:55	20:46	20:36	20:28
15	28:15	26:17	24:43	23:19	22:00	21:22	20:44	20:05	19:57	19:49	19:40	19:31
16	27:41	25:45	24:08	22:44	21:23	20:43	20:03	19:22	19:15	19:06	18:58	18:49
17	27:28	25:36	23:57	22:29	21:07	20:25	19:42	18:58	18:49	18:40	18:32	18:22
18	27:40	25:44	24:04	22:36	21:12	20:27	19:40	18:51	18:40	18:31	18:22	18:11
19	28:02	26:05	24:26	22:57	21:30	20:44	19:53	18:59	18:47	18:36	18:26	18:14
20	28:30	26:32	24:54	23:26	21:57	21:10	20:17	19:19	19:05	18:53	18:42	18:28
21	28:57	27:00	25:23	23:56	22:26	21:39	20:44	19:44	19:30	19:17	19:04	18:48
22	29:20	27:24	25:48	24:21	22:50	22:04	21:10	20:10	19:55	19:41	19:28	19:11
23	29:36	27:42	26:07	24:41	23:11	22:26	21:33	20:33	20:18	20:05	19:51	19:33
24	29:51	27:59	26:23	24:57	23:28	22:43	21:52	20:54	20:40	20:26	20:12	19:55

AGE ↓	MALE Centile ↙ ↘											
	90th	91st	92nd	93rd	94th	95th	96th	97th	98th	99th	99.5th	99.9th
12	22:29	22:17	22:04	21:50	21:36	21:19	21:00	20:37	20:09	19:32	18:57	17:57
13	21:22	21:11	20:59	20:47	20:34	20:18	20:03	19:42	19:17	18:44	18:12	17:20
14	20:19	20:08	19:58	19:47	19:35	19:21	19:08	18:50	18:28	17:59	17:31	16:47
15	19:23	19:13	19:04	18:54	18:43	18:31	18:20	18:05	17:46	17:21	16:57	16:18
16	18:41	18:31	18:22	18:13	18:03	17:52	17:42	17:29	17:13	16:50	16:29	15:55
17	18:14	18:04	17:54	17:45	17:35	17:25	17:14	17:02	16:47	16:26	16:08	15:37
18	18:01	17:51	17:40	17:29	17:19	17:08	16:57	16:44	16:28	16:08	15:52	15:22
19	18:02	17:51	17:37	17:24	17:12	16:59	16:46	16:31	16:14	15:54	15:39	15:08
20	18:14	18:01	17:45	17:29	17:14	16:57	16:41	16:24	16:05	15:43	15:26	14:53
21	18:33	18:18	18:00	17:40	17:21	17:01	16:42	16:22	15:59	15:34	15:15	14:38
22	18:53	18:37	18:17	17:55	17:33	17:09	16:47	16:23	15:57	15:28	15:05	14:22
23	19:15	18:57	18:37	18:13	17:48	17:21	16:56	16:28	15:59	15:26	14:59	14:10
24	19:37	19:18	18:58	18:35	18:07	17:39	17:11	16:39	16:07	15:29	14:58	14:03

Table 5iii   Adult
Time (in Minutes:Seconds) for Selected Centiles

AGE ↓	↙ MALE Centile ↘											
	30th	40th	50th	60th	70th	75th	80th	85th	86th	87th	88th	89th
25	30:05	28:14	26:38	25:11	23:44	22:59	22:07	21:10	20:57	20:44	20:30	20:13
26	30:20	28:29	26:53	25:26	23:58	23:12	22:21	21:24	21:12	20:58	20:45	20:29
27	30:34	28:42	27:06	25:38	24:11	23:25	22:33	21:36	21:24	21:11	20:57	20:42
28	30:47	28:54	27:17	25:50	24:22	23:35	22:43	21:46	21:34	21:21	21:08	20:52
29	30:57	29:03	27:26	25:58	24:30	23:43	22:50	21:53	21:41	21:28	21:14	20:59
30	31:04	29:09	27:32	26:04	24:35	23:48	22:55	21:57	21:45	21:32	21:18	21:03
31	31:07	29:12	27:36	26:07	24:38	23:51	22:59	22:00	21:48	21:34	21:20	21:06
32	31:09	29:14	27:39	26:08	24:40	23:53	23:01	22:03	21:51	21:37	21:23	21:09
33	31:12	29:16	27:41	26:09	24:42	23:55	23:03	22:05	21:53	21:40	21:26	21:12
34	31:17	29:20	27:43	26:10	24:44	23:57	23:06	22:09	21:57	21:44	21:31	21:16
35	31:24	29:25	27:46	26:13	24:46	24:00	23:09	22:14	22:01	21:49	21:36	21:22
36	31:31	29:29	27:49	26:16	24:50	24:03	23:13	22:18	22:06	21:54	21:41	21:27
37	31:36	29:32	27:51	26:19	24:53	24:06	23:16	22:21	22:08	21:57	21:44	21:30
38	31:41	29:36	27:55	26:23	24:56	24:09	23:18	22:23	22:10	21:58	21:46	21:32
39	31:45	29:40	27:58	26:26	24:58	24:11	23:20	22:23	22:10	21:58	21:46	21:32

AGE ↓	↙ MALE Centile ↘											
	90th	91st	92nd	93rd	94th	95th	96th	97th	98th	99th	99.5th	99.9th
25	19:56	19:38	19:18	18:56	18:27	17:59	17:30	16:55	16:19	15:37	15:03	14:02
26	20:13	19:55	19:36	19:15	18:48	18:20	17:50	17:13	16:34	15:48	15:12	14:08
27	20:27	20:09	19:52	19:32	19:06	18:39	18:09	17:31	16:49	16:01	15:25	14:18
28	20:38	20:21	20:04	19:45	19:22	18:56	18:27	17:48	17:04	16:13	15:37	14:30
29	20:46	20:29	20:13	19:53	19:32	19:07	18:39	18:02	17:18	16:23	15:47	14:41
30	20:50	20:34	20:17	19:58	19:39	19:15	18:48	18:13	17:29	16:32	15:53	14:50
31	20:53	20:37	20:21	20:01	19:43	19:19	18:53	18:21	17:38	16:40	15:58	14:58
32	20:56	20:40	20:24	20:04	19:46	19:23	18:57	18:26	17:46	16:48	16:03	15:06
33	20:58	20:43	20:27	20:08	19:49	19:26	19:00	18:32	17:53	16:56	16:09	15:16
34	21:02	20:47	20:31	20:12	19:53	19:30	19:05	18:37	18:00	17:05	16:17	15:27
35	21:08	20:52	20:37	20:18	19:58	19:36	19:10	18:43	18:07	17:13	16:28	15:37
36	21:12	20:57	20:42	20:23	20:03	19:41	19:15	18:47	18:12	17:20	16:37	15:44
37	21:15	21:00	20:44	20:26	20:06	19:43	19:19	18:50	18:16	17:24	16:45	15:48
38	21:17	21:02	20:46	20:28	20:08	19:46	19:22	18:52	18:18	17:28	16:51	15:48
39	21:17	21:02	20:46	20:27	20:08	19:47	19:24	18:54	18:19	17:31	16:55	15:48

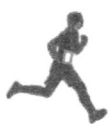

MALE Ages 40-54 **MALE Ages 40-54**

Table 5iv   Early Masters
Time (in Minutes:Seconds) for Selected Centiles

AGE ↓	MALE Centile ↙ ↘											
	30th	40th	50th	60th	70th	75th	80th	85th	86th	87th	88th	89th
40	31:51	29:45	28:03	26:30	25:00	24:13	23:21	22:23	22:11	21:58	21:46	21:32
41	32:01	29:53	28:09	26:34	25:02	24:15	23:23	22:24	22:12	21:59	21:46	21:32
42	32:14	30:03	28:17	26:39	25:05	24:17	23:25	22:26	22:13	22:01	21:48	21:33
43	32:36	30:18	28:27	26:46	25:10	24:21	23:29	22:29	22:17	22:04	21:51	21:36
44	33:07	30:36	28:39	26:56	25:16	24:26	23:34	22:34	22:21	22:08	21:54	21:40
45	33:36	30:57	28:52	27:06	25:24	24:34	23:40	22:40	22:27	22:14	22:00	21:46
46	34:48	31:22	29:09	27:19	25:34	24:43	23:47	22:48	22:34	22:21	22:07	21:53
47	35:54	31:48	29:27	27:33	25:45	24:53	23:56	22:56	22:42	22:29	22:15	22:00
48	37:15	32:27	29:50	27:49	25:58	25:05	24:06	23:05	22:51	22:38	22:24	22:09
49	39:39	33:10	30:18	28:09	26:13	25:18	24:18	23:15	23:02	22:49	22:35	22:19
50	44:33	34:12	30:50	28:34	26:32	25:33	24:33	23:28	23:15	23:01	22:47	22:31
51	53:11	36:22	31:47	29:05	26:57	25:54	24:52	23:44	23:31	23:16	23:01	22:46
52	<60	39:29	32:55	29:37	27:23	26:17	25:12	24:02	23:48	23:33	23:17	23:01
53	<60	44:35	34:30	30:19	27:56	26:47	25:38	24:25	24:10	23:53	23:36	23:20
54	<60	52:56	36:45	31:16	28:37	27:22	26:09	24:52	24:35	24:18	24:00	23:42

AGE ↓	MALE Centile ↙ ↘											
	90th	91st	92nd	93rd	94th	95th	96th	97th	98th	99th	99.5th	99.9th
40	21:17	21:02	20:45	20:27	20:08	19:47	19:25	18:55	18:20	17:33	16:58	15:49
41	21:16	21:02	20:45	20:27	20:09	19:48	19:26	18:56	18:22	17:37	17:01	15:53
42	21:18	21:02	20:46	20:28	20:10	19:50	19:28	18:59	18:25	17:41	17:05	15:59
43	21:21	21:05	20:49	20:31	20:13	19:53	19:31	19:02	18:29	17:46	17:11	16:06
44	21:25	21:09	20:53	20:35	20:16	19:57	19:34	19:06	18:35	17:51	17:16	16:14
45	21:30	21:14	20:58	20:39	20:19	20:00	19:37	19:11	18:40	17:57	17:23	16:21
46	21:37	21:21	21:04	20:45	20:25	20:06	19:42	19:17	18:46	18:04	17:30	16:28
47	21:45	21:29	21:12	20:52	20:32	20:13	19:49	19:24	18:54	18:10	17:37	16:34
48	21:54	21:38	21:20	21:01	20:41	20:21	19:57	19:32	19:01	18:18	17:44	16:42
49	22:04	21:48	21:30	21:12	20:52	20:31	20:06	19:41	19:09	18:25	17:51	16:50
50	22:16	21:59	21:42	21:23	21:03	20:42	20:17	19:51	19:18	18:33	17:59	16:59
51	22:30	22:12	21:55	21:36	21:16	20:54	20:28	20:02	19:27	18:41	18:08	17:09
52	22:44	22:27	22:09	21:50	21:29	21:06	20:40	20:12	19:37	18:50	18:18	17:19
53	23:02	22:45	22:26	22:05	21:44	21:20	20:53	20:24	19:49	19:00	18:28	17:29
54	23:24	23:06	22:45	22:24	22:01	21:37	21:09	20:38	20:02	19:12	18:38	17:39

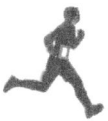

Table 5v   Middle Masters
Time (in Minutes:Seconds) for Selected Centiles

AGE ↓	MALE Centile											
	30th	40th	50th	60th	70th	75th	80th	85th	86th	87th	88th	89th
55	---	<60	39:59	32:33	29:24	28:02	26:43	25:21	25:03	24:44	24:25	24:07
56	---	<60	44:36	35:16	30:14	28:43	27:17	25:50	25:31	25:11	24:51	24:32
57	---	<60	51:26	38:29	31:05	29:23	27:50	26:18	25:59	25:38	25:17	24:57
58	---	---	<60	43:10	32:14	30:08	28:26	26:48	26:28	26:06	25:45	25:23
59	---	---	<60	47:43	33:13	30:58	29:03	27:18	26:57	26:34	26:13	25:50
60	---	---	<60	52:35	34:59	31:53	29:45	27:49	27:26	27:03	26:40	26:16
61	---	---	<60	57:39	38:09	33:42	30:36	28:25	28:01	27:36	27:12	26:47
62	---	---	---	<60	42:22	35:35	31:34	29:06	28:38	28:12	27:47	27:20
63	---	---	---	<60	47:27	38:24	33:02	29:57	29:25	28:56	28:29	27:58
64	---	---	---	<60	54:10	41:47	34:10	30:53	30:15	29:42	29:12	28:38
65	---	---	---	---	<60	45:26	35:59	32:01	31:14	30:35	30:00	29:21
66	---	---	---	---	<60	49:37	39:50	33:32	32:24	31:36	30:54	30:11
67	---	---	---	---	<60	54:28	44:10	34:37	33:39	32:45	31:54	31:04
68	---	---	---	---	---	<60	48:42	36:25	35:27	34:12	33:05	32:05
69	---	---	---	---	---	<60	53:49	38:00	37:04	35:31	34:11	33:11

AGE ↓	MALE Centile											
	90th	91st	92nd	93rd	94th	95th	96th	97th	98th	99th	99.5th	99.9th
55	23:46	23:28	23:06	22:43	22:20	21:55	21:26	20:53	20:18	19:26	18:50	17:48
56	24:10	23:50	23:26	23:02	22:39	22:13	21:43	21:09	20:34	19:41	19:01	18:00
57	24:33	24:12	23:46	23:22	22:58	22:32	22:00	21:26	20:50	19:57	19:14	18:13
58	24:59	24:35	24:08	23:43	23:18	22:53	22:20	21:45	21:08	20:14	19:29	18:27
59	25:24	24:58	24:31	24:05	23:40	23:13	22:40	22:04	21:25	20:32	19:48	18:44
60	25:50	25:23	24:54	24:28	24:01	23:33	22:59	22:22	21:41	20:50	20:07	18:59
61	26:20	25:52	25:23	24:54	24:25	23:55	23:21	22:42	22:00	21:07	20:24	19:11
62	26:53	26:24	25:54	25:23	24:51	24:18	23:44	23:04	22:18	21:23	20:39	19:21
63	27:29	27:00	26:28	25:53	25:19	24:43	24:09	23:25	22:37	21:37	20:52	19:33
64	28:07	27:36	27:01	26:24	25:47	25:08	24:32	23:46	22:54	21:51	21:02	19:44
65	28:47	28:13	27:36	26:55	26:16	25:36	24:57	24:08	23:13	22:06	21:10	19:58
66	29:31	28:53	28:11	27:28	26:47	26:06	25:23	24:32	23:33	22:24	21:23	20:15
67	30:16	29:33	28:47	28:01	27:19	26:35	25:49	24:55	23:54	22:45	21:41	20:36
68	31:08	30:19	29:29	28:39	27:54	27:05	26:16	25:20	24:18	23:11	22:05	20:58
69	32:05	31:09	30:16	29:20	28:32	27:38	26:46	25:48	24:45	23:39	22:32	21:21

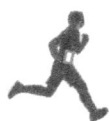

MALE Ages 70-89   **MALE Ages 70-89**

Table 5vi   Later Masters
Time (in Minutes:Seconds) for Selected Centiles

AGE ↓	↙ MALE Centile ↘											
	30th	40th	50th	60th	70th	75th	80th	85th	86th	87th	88th	89th
70	---	---	---	---	---	<60	59:36	40:18	39:37	37:33	35:55	34:33
71	---	---	---	---	---	---	<60	44:36	42:45	40:00	37:59	36:15
72	---	---	---	---	---	---	<60	51:35	46:50	43:03	40:35	37:56
73	---	---	---	---	---	---	---	<60	52:18	47:08	44:01	41:10
74	---	---	---	---	---	---	---	<60	59:54	52:37	48:31	44:51
75	---	---	---	---	---	---	---	---	---	<60	54:39	49:15
76	---	---	---	---	---	---	---	---	---	---	<60	54:49
77	---	---	---	---	---	---	---	---	---	---	---	<60
78	---	---	---	---	---	---	---	---	---	---	---	---
79	---	---	---	---	---	---	---	---	---	---	---	---

AGE ↓	↙ MALE Centile ↘											
	90th	91st	92nd	93rd	94th	95th	96th	97th	98th	99th	99.5th	99.9th
70	33:16	32:14	31:15	30:12	29:17	28:16	27:20	26:19	25:15	24:07	23:01	21:42
71	34:45	33:34	32:26	31:16	30:13	29:04	28:03	26:58	25:50	24:37	23:32	22:01
72	36:22	34:57	33:45	32:23	31:12	29:55	28:48	27:38	26:27	25:06	24:00	22:12
73	39:11	37:19	35:40	33:58	32:31	30:59	29:44	28:27	27:10	25:36	24:25	22:22
74	42:21	39:45	36:49	35:05	33:30	32:04	30:43	29:21	27:58	26:11	24:53	22:41
75	45:40	42:01	39:05	36:29	34:41	33:04	31:43	30:15	28:45	26:50	25:26	23:07
76	49:25	44:16	42:15	39:36	36:54	34:50	33:04	31:15	29:38	27:36	26:09	23:39
77	53:39	46:27	45:47	42:47	39:10	36:14	34:01	32:22	30:38	28:26	26:56	24:24
78	---	<60	49:47	46:33	41:54	38:37	35:46	33:53	31:51	29:27	27:53	25:12
79	---	<60	54:30	51:10	45:16	41:55	38:18	35:55	33:17	30:40	28:57	25:53
80	---	---	<60	57:00	49:29	47:03	41:34	38:34	34:59	31:55	29:58	26:17
81	---	---	---	---	<60	55:05	46:12	42:02	37:14	33:19	31:03	26:42
82	---	---	---	---	---	<60	52:49	45:34	40:00	34:56	32:13	27:17
83	---	---	---	---	---	---	<60	49:27	43:53	36:43	33:29	27:58
84	---	---	---	---	---	---	<60	53:44	48:32	38:46	35:00	29:03
85	---	---	---	---	---	---	---	<60	53:52	41:05	36:52	30:45
86	---	---	---	---	---	---	---	<60	57:08	43:42	39:05	32:53
87	---	---	---	---	---	---	---	<60	58:30	45:54	41:17	34:47
88	---	---	---	---	---	---	---	<60	57:39	47:47	43:35	36:40
89	---	---	---	---	---	---	---	---	<60	49:15	45:59	38:29

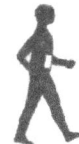

THE AUTHOR

David P. Dyer received his Ph.D. from The Johns Hopkins University and was a post-doctoral fellow in Statistics and Biomathematics at North Carolina State University. Employed for thirty-seven years as an industrial statistician and business analyst, his professional interests include data analytics, efficiency metrics, process design, economic optimization, experimental design, sampling, and market analysis.

David's personal interests include sports math, running and racing, nine grandchildren, and his lovely wife, Kathy Mae

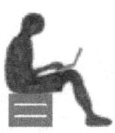

Bibliography

Davis, John. (2015). *How to Use Age Grade Calculators Effectively*, unnersconnect.net/masters-running/age-grading/

Fair, Ray C. (1994). How Fast Do Old Men Slow Down? *The Review of Economics and Statistics 76*: 103-118

Fair, Ray C. (2007). Estimated Age Effects in Athletic Events and Chess, *Experimental Aging Research, 33*: 37-57

Grubb, Howard. (1998). Models for comparing athletic performances, *The Statistician, 47*: 509-521

Hreljac, Alan, Daryl Parker, Roberto Quintana, Estelle Abdala, Kyle Patterson, Mitell Sison. (2002). Energetics and Perceived Exertion of Low Speed Running and High Speed Walking, *Physical Education and Sport Vol. 1, No. 9*:27-37

Jones, Alan (2015). *Age Grading Running Races*, www.runscore.com/Alan/AgeGrade.html

Long, Leroy and Manoj Srinivasan. (2013). Walking, Running, and Resting under Time, Distance, and Average Speed Constraints: Optimality of Walk—Run—Rest Mixtures, *J R Soc. Interface 10*: 20120980

Minetti, Alberto E., Lorenzo Boldrini, Laura Brusamolin, Paola Zamparo, and Tom McKee. (2003). A Feedback-controlled Treadmill (Treadmill-on-demand) and the Spontaneous Speed of Walking and Running in Humans, *J Appl Physiol 95*:838-843.

Reece, Robert James, and Christine Fennessy. (2014). How the World Record Affected Age-Graded Percentages, *Runner's World October*.

Savitzky, A., and M.J.E. Golay. (1964). Smoothing and Differentiation of Data by Simplified Least Squares Procedures, *Anal. Chem. 36*: 1627-1639

Schafer, Ronald A., (2011). What is a Savitzky-Golay Filter?, *IEEE Signal Processing Magazine, July*: 111-117

Schoonjans, Frank, Dirk De Bacquer, and Pirmin Schmid. (2011). Estimation of Population Percentiles, *Epidemiology 22(5)*:750-751

Sterken, Elmer. (2003). From the Cradle to the Grave: How Fast Can We Run?, *Journal of Sports Sciences, 21*:479-491